Dr. Hur___
Rec___
Optimum ___ealth

A Nutritional Approach to Overall Wellness and Detoxification of the Body

Elizabeth Huntley, PhD

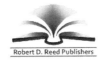

Robert D. Reed Publishers

Robert D. Reed Publishers • Bandon, Oregon

Robert D. Reed Publishers
P.O. Box 1992
Bandon, OR 97411
Phone: 541-347-9882; Fax: -9883
E-mail: 4bobreed@msn.com
Website: www.rdrpublishers.com

Editor: Jessica Bryan, www.oregoneditor.wordpress.com
Cover Design: David Dees, www.DDees.com
Interior Design: Susan Leonard

Soft cover ISBN: 978-1-944297-14-5
eBook ISBN: 978-1-944297-13-8
Library of Congress Control Number: 2016958161

DISCLAIMER: The information contained herein is intended to be of a general educational nature and does not constitute medical, legal, or other professional advice for any specific individual or situation. It is not to be used as the sole means of diagnosis, prescription, or treatment of any health disorder. The author and publisher are in no way liable for any misuse of the material, and readers are encouraged to see a medical doctor or other professional for any illness or suspected illness.

Designed and Formatted in the United States of America

Never accept what anyone else tells you to believe. Find the truth for yourself and contribute what you can to the welfare of the world.

– Elizabeth Huntley, PhD

Acknowledgments

With loving gratitude to:
Takana A. Gottschalk and Michael R. Moore for their help
in writing this book and testing the recipes

Jessica Bryan, the editor who prepared the manuscript
for publication.
www.oregoneditor.wordpress.com

David Dees, for his beautiful cover design
www.DDees.com

and

Anne apRoberts, Abbess of the Order of the Trees,
for her kindness and support
www.eloinforest.org

Contents

Foreword

by Michael Moore

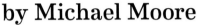

first met Elizabeth Huntley in 1990. I was visiting a friend in Los Angeles for spring break. He introduced me to Elizabeth because he was working for her at the time. He told me many stories about how she had helped hundreds of people with her nutritional counseling. He had observed her over the course of almost a year and had seen hundreds of successes occur. It stuck in my mind. I remembered it. Four years later, I moved to Los Angeles myself. I told my friend I was really tired of being sick all the time. I said I was interested in locating her, and I asked him if he thought she could help me. He told me he felt certain she could. I, like Elizabeth, had been sickly my whole life and didn't know why.

We located her, and I set up an appointment for nutritional counseling. She tested me with her radionics machine and told me that my immune system was extremely suppressed. This was probably why I had been so sickly my whole life. I asked her if we could fix it and she said we could. All I had to do was follow the nutritional program and the diet. I was very motivated because was tired of being sick. So, I followed her recommendations. I felt better and better as the weeks and months went by. I loved the work she was doing so much that I started working as her receptionist.

This was the beginning of more than a decade of collaboration between us. I continued to use her nutritional program as part of my healing process. It wasn't the only part, but it was significant. After several years on the nutritional program, Elizabeth discovered extremely high readings of mercury in my body. We began to realize this was likely the source of my lifelong health problems. After some research, I realized that I had been poisoned by mercury when I was in utero, before I was even born. My mother had many mercury amalgam fillings during her pregnancy with my brother and me. My brother was born first, and during that pregnancy the leaking of her fillings started. When she was pregnant with me, I received the full force of the mercury poisoning.

I realized that we both needed to get the mercury out of our bodies. I had my mother go to a dentist who specialized in mercury filling removal. Thus, we began a long journey of detoxification. After many years, we are both free of mercury. My current health and the way I feel is nothing like it was for the first part of my life. I actually have the energy to do things, and I am not eternally ill.

I credit Elizabeth with helping me discover the problem and detoxify the mercury, and also with teaching me the basics of healthy living. She taught me to take responsibility for my life, including what I put in my mouth. I have come to realize that many of the health problems people have are directly related to what they put in their mouths. Many people eat garbage and pay dearly for it. So, I embarked on a new chapter of my life in which I knew and understood what healthy foods are, where to get them, and how to prepare them. I worked with Elizabeth for many years managing her office and her finances, and assisting her in her research. What I learned was invaluable.

Elizabeth used a radionics device in her nutritional practice. She did not use the device to broadcast energy to her clients. Instead, she used it to test for imbalances in their electromagnetic field. Every person's body is surrounded by an electromagnetic field, and there is a significant amount of information available in this area. Elizabeth used a process that she developed for combing through all of this information in order to find problems. Sometimes, these problems would be caused by a pathogen. Other times they would be caused by deficiencies in the person's body related to our poor modern diet; and, finally, sometimes their problems were emotional. When the client was having emotional issues, usually they were helped significantly just by having these issues pointed out to them.

However, as far as pathogens and deficiencies, Elizabeth's solution was the recommendation of specific nutritional supplements. She primarily used Standard Process Labs supplements because of their high quality and effectiveness. She also used an entire array of other supplements that she had found to be useful over the years. She would usually give dietary recommendations to help people avoid foods that were bad for them, and direct them to seek foods that were good for them. Improving diet alone goes a long way towards resolving these deficiencies, but, often, the deficiencies were so deep that nutritional supplements sped up the process dramatically.

In observing many clients who were on her nutritional program, I began to realize there was only one requirement for them to improve or get well, and that was to simply follow the program. If they received her instructions and continued to eat garbage and not take their supplements, they would not get better. However, if they simply followed her instructions, they got better. It was a very rewarding process to witness. It also taught me much about the meaning of personal responsibility. We are all individually responsible for the quality of our lives, and diet is simply one area in which this truth shines through.

I am delighted that these lovely people have come together to bring this book to reality. Elizabeth is a special person. She doesn't fit neatly into the compartments that society expects. She is truly a rebel, but not a "Rebel Without a Cause." Her cause is to bring knowledge and healing to others. Her cause is to assist others in taking responsibility for their health. Only then, when this responsibility is present, can vibrant health begin to show up. Thank you, Elizabeth, for taking a stand for all of us. Your work has truly made a difference in this world.

With much love,
Michael Moore

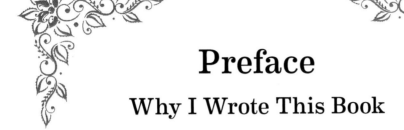

Preface
Why I Wrote This Book

When I was a child, the dream came every night. I was floating in a bag of fluid. It was warm and comfortable there, but, from the edge of the bag, I could feel something poisonous seeping in to my space. I knew if it all came into my body, it would kill me. I was frightened, but there was nothing I could do. I was helpless against this deadly poison. In my dream, I was, in fact, an embryo.

I didn't think of this as a nightmare. I just thought, *this is my peculiar dream*, and didn't try to do anything about it. Although I had heard my father tell my mother (after I was supposedly asleep) that he hadn't set any money aside for my college education because I probably wouldn't live that long, I did make it through my junior year of high school and got accepted to college a year early. When I got away from home, I no longer had the dream, but every time I came back to visit it would recur.

As an adult, exploring alternative health care, I became interested in hair analyses and had one done. Arsenic showed up as a major problem in my body. Trying to understand how this happened, I asked my father if we kept any poisons containing arsenic around the house when I was young. He became quite angry and told me not to call him any more.

After my mother told me that my father had begged her to have an abortion every time she got pregnant, I started to put the story together. (My mother was Catholic and said she thought she would go to hell if she acceded to my father's requests.)

My father was our family doctor until I was a teenager and could go to Public Health Clinics. He used to give my mother pills he thought she needed. I suspect he thought she needed arsenic to cause an abortion. It didn't work.

Whatever the reason, I was quite sickly as a child. I couldn't walk until I was two years old. My mother had starved herself when she was pregnant, accepting some bad advice that made her think she would have smaller babies and thus fewer problems with delivery that way. Her response to my problem with walking was to think that I was too fat. So she put me on a starvation diet. I was finally able to walk, but continued to be sickly. Decades later, I had X-rays from a chiropractor, who said, "Oh, that deformed hip joint is probably congenital."

I was never able to participate in the physical activities of most children my age—I gave that up early on. But by the time I went to college at 17, it was clear that I would have some difficulty even participating in the intellectual life that had become my refuge. I was found to have a heart murmur, and my resistance to infections was so low that I was routinely in the school infirmary for a few days every two weeks when the latest virus came through.

This was long before the label of "chronic fatigue syndrome" became popular. At that time, I was just labeled "frail" and told not to do much activity. My parents had done their best to raise me in good health, applying the knowledge they had acquired in those days of "better living through chemistry!" We ate frozen vegetables, Velveeta cheese, Spam, margarine, and other "superior, modern foods." One of my memories of childhood was of being allowed to break the color capsule that came in the white margarine and knead it in to give the margarine a cheerful yellow color. As an adult, it came to my attention that the capsule contained "butter yellow," a dye that is now sometimes used in research laboratories to induce cancer in rats, because it is a fairly effective carcinogen.

My father, being a medical doctor, tried to help me by testing out the latest drugs on my symptoms: constant colds, allergies, fatigue, and digestive problems. I was given penicillin lozenges (sweetened with sugar) to suck on like candy. I also recall being given a Milltown (the first tranquilizer) as a teenager for a headache. It worked—I slept for two days and woke up without the headache!

Upon entering college, I encountered some revelations that changed my attitude toward all this. First of all, I developed friends who lived on "health foods." I found that there was such a thing as whole-wheat flour—I'd never seen anything but the bleached variety before. The amazing thing was that the food they ate tasted good! In fact, it had a lot more flavor than what I had been eating.

Secondly, I learned there were people who were known as "nutritionists," and they actually helped people get healthier by monitoring their diet and giving them nutritional supplements. I thought I'd better find out something about this, so I studied Adelle Davis and the few other authors available at that point.

Although academically I was seduced into the "basic sciences"—physics as an undergraduate, a master's degree in biology, and a PhD in biological and medical sciences—I kept up my personal study of nutrition and tried to haul myself up by my bootstraps. I was not solely satisfied by a career as a research scientist. I also wanted to raise children. By the time my daughter was born, I was growing some of our own vegetables in an organic garden, baking all our bread, and keeping my family on a diet of primarily organically grown food, in addition to holding down part-time research jobs, including research on nutrition.

Unfortunately, the birth of my first child led to a setback in my physical condition. A modern HMO, with the latest technology and computerized record keeping, monitored my pregnancy. However, the computer somehow lost my blood tests, so it wasn't found that I was severely anemic until I was eight months pregnant. This led to some major problems, culminating in an emergency C-section. Neither my daughter nor I recovered well. I developed more serious allergies. She did well, at first, but then she developed chronic ear infections in her second year and actually lost two pounds between her first and second birthdays, apparently due to the fact that the heavy doses of antibiotics and antihistamines (the medical solution to the ear problems) were destroying her appetite.

In desperation, I looked for any help I could get in solving her problems. I found the last licensed naturopathic physician in northern Florida and sought advice from him. Dr. Hardy was 85 years old at the time, had all his own hair and all his own teeth, got up at 6:00 a.m., and worked in his garden until noon. Then he cleaned up and saw patients until 10:00 p.m. This was a pretty good recommendation for him, but when I saw him testing my daughter by putting litmus paper in her mouth and looking for spots in her iris, I thought: *This guy is a quack for sure, but I'm desperate enough to give it a try.*

The results of the supplements he gave her were nothing short of miraculous. The second night after starting them, my daughter, who had to be coaxed to eat *anything*, ate two adult-sized plates of food at dinner and five bananas before bedtime! Within three weeks, she was off drugs and she had *no* more ear infections.

I was in shock. I went back to the naturopath and demanded to know why I, who had all this academic training in physiology and biochemistry, who had done research in nutrition, who had read every book I could find on nutrition—why I didn't know any of this. Why, with all this education, didn't I understand the first thing about how he had been able to work this miracle? How could I have read the labels on the bottles of supplements he had given me and not have the faintest idea what they did or why.

Dr. Hardy introduced me to the shocking condition of health care in this country: the suppression of knowledge and the perversion of truth for profit. The corruption of the healing arts has become an *industry* that supports the practice of removing and replacing diseased hearts at the cost of hundreds of thousands of dollars and produces devastating results to the body so mistreated, but that attempts to ban from the public the knowledge of how to prevent the heart from becoming diseased. He educated me with regard to the laws that allow the Food and Drug Administration to operate under the policy that "Information given to the physician must be true and not misrepresent. Information given to the general public, however, must conform to the consensus of medical opinion, whether that be true or false" (from legislation establishing the FDA in 1938).

This experience started my quest for data and understanding. It led to starting my own nutritional practice forty years ago, and it led to the research that resulted in this book. What I want to do in this book is give you tools and understanding that will help you find out the truth about your body for yourself and attain health, even immortality!

Elizabeth Huntley, PhD
Medford, Oregon, 2017

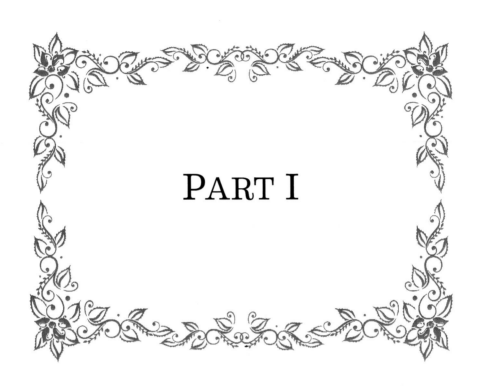

PART I

1

The Nutritionist's Heritage

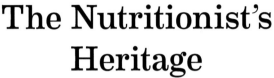

n this country, we have professionals who are called "MDs," which stands for "Medical Doctors." These people have a powerful influence over our lives. Through the American Medical Association (AMA), they control what actions we can legally take to help ourselves when we are ill, and a great deal of the information we can obtain about staying healthy. In some countries (and in past times, in this country), this type of physician did not have the same power or monopoly.

There are five types of physicians in common practice in developed countries:

1. The Allopathic Physician (*allo*, meaning against, and *path*, meaning disease). The allopath (also known as a medical doctor or MD) uses surgery and substances that fight disease or the symptoms of disease. Usually, this means drugs that either kill off harmful organisms or suppress the symptoms of the affliction.

2. The Homeopathic Physician (*homeo*, meaning like, therefore "like the disease"). The homeopath works in just the opposite way. He gives the patient a minute quantity of a substance that, if given in a large dose, would produce the same symptoms as the disease produces. For example, if a person has a fever, the homeopath would give a tiny quantity of a substance that

causes fevers. Because the body is a homeostatic system (meaning it is designed to keep itself in balance), it will react against the intruding foreign substance and will bring the fever down. A good homeopath can work miracles.

3. Doctors of Chiropractic (or DC) study structural misalignment and how to correct it. Some chiropractors work primarily with structure; others employ a wide variety of holistic and other modalities to help their patients achieve maximum health and mobility. Chiropractic is based on the principle that the body can heal itself when the skeletal system is correctly aligned and the nervous system is functioning properly. Chiropractic treatment is non-invasive and carries none of the risks of surgery or pharmaceutical drugs.

4. Originating around 100 B.C., acupuncture is a key component of traditional Chinese medicine involving thin needles that are inserted into the body at specific acupuncture points. It can also be associated with the application of heat, pressure or laser light. Acupuncture is commonly used for pain relief and other conditions. This type of treatment has gained a lot of attention and respect in Western countries during the past 50 years because of its unique effectiveness and safety.

5. The Naturopathic Physician (Doctor of Naturopathy) practices natural healing of disease. This physician uses diet or special foods, herbs, vitamins, and other healing modalities to help the body repair itself. Many naturopathic physicians also use natural, non-invasive methods of diagnosis, such as observation, iridology, and listening to the symptoms of the patient in order to diagnose health problems.

These different types of physicians, with their different approaches to healing, may be considered to complement each other, because one approach might more successful in an individual case than another. Unfortunately, this differential utilization of skills has not been allowed to take its normal course in this country.

In the early 1900s, John D. Rockefeller, Sr. decided to use much of his amassed fortune for philanthropy (for perhaps not so philanthropic reasons. See *The Rockefeller File*.) His foundation donated huge sums to a select number of medical schools on the condition that they stop teaching homeopathy and teach only allopathic medicine instead. The net result of this "philanthropy" was that almost two-thirds of the alternative medicine schools closed down over the next few decades, starved for funds, and that allopaths became the primarily accepted type of physician. In more recent years, there has been a shift back to alternative practitioners such as homeopaths, chiropractors, and naturopaths.

One rationale for this might be that the Rockefeller holdings included major drug firms, and homeopaths use only minute quantities of drugs. But an ironic note is that John D. Sr. would not allow an allopath near him. His doctor was always a homeopath!

Further steps in the monopolizing of medical care were taken by the establishment of intensive lobbying practices by the AMA, with the result that homeopaths and naturopaths were widely regarded as quacks, although this has changed in recent years. This is in addition to the intense campaign that the AMA has carried on against chiropractors. See *Are You a Target for Elimination?*

Medical doctors have become the primary medical resource for a large majority of the American public, especially with the passage of the Affordable Care Act. They have succeeded in treating contagious diseases through the use of inoculations and antibiotics, but now that contagious diseases are no longer a major medical problem in this country, they have turned their attention to developing more and more pharmaceutical drugs for degenerative diseases such as arthritis, heart disease, and cancer. Of course, many of these new drugs cause us more trouble than they help. Just watch the advertisements on television that talk about how great these drugs are, and then also warn us that they "might" cause death and other horrible health problems. Even more bizarre, the ads promoting these products are often followed up by offers from law firms to sue the drug companies for the trouble their "great" medications have caused!

By using the term "degenerative," it is obvious that these diseases indicate a lack of balance in the body. The other schools of medicine specifically work to bring the body back into a balance. The allopath does not. So the response of someone who works "against disease" becomes limited, and actually ludicrous, at times, in dealing with degenerative diseases, such as the idea that a diseased heart should be removed and replaced with an artificial one.

Additional disciplines have arisen in reaction to the suppression of natural healing, one of which is the "nutritional consultant." Widely ignored by the medical establishment—and not licensed in many states because nobody can agree on what they are supposed to do—they use natural substances such as foods, herbs, and vitamins, the sale of which is not restricted. Not being licensed physicians, they are not allowed by law to diagnose or tell their clients what is wrong with them, nor are they allowed to advise their clients to stop taking pharmaceutical medications. There is no standardization of their discipline, and we find extremely conflicting materials being put out on prevention and treatment of diseases by nutritional methods. Some of this may be due to the fact that schools of nutrition at major universities are funded by some of the big food manufacturing companies, who are far more concerned with profit than health.

Nutritionists carry a great responsibility. She must largely educate herself, for if she goes to a school of nutrition, she may be educated into the belief that white sugar is a "valuable health food"—in the words of a former dean of the school of nutrition of one of the most prestigious universities in the country. She must realize that she is fighting against a great deal of advertising that says food is "sexy" or that only taste counts. She holds the future generations of this country in her hands, because a malnourished people become easy prey for subversion and dictators.

My academic training includes a PhD in Biological and Medical Sciences, but much of what I've learned about nutrition comes from the writings of Dr. Royal Lee, the founder of Standard Process Labs, the oldest supplement company in the country. Dr. Lee recognized that there are many micronutrients the body needs to be healthy. He also realized that natural foods are the best form to get them in, so he developed a line of supplements that are extracts of organically grown whole foods. I recommended these supplements for many years in my private practice as a nutritionist.

One of the most important results to come out of my research is that each individual is different from everyone else. There is no universal diet that is going to make everybody healthy. There are some basic concepts about diet that are common to most people, and there are some basic principles of "body care." But *you* have to find the right diet, the right system for *you*. I will give you all the help I can.

This is a great exploratory adventure that I have been on for some decades, I welcome your company.

2

Chemicals Don't Cure

ne of the tragedies of the imbalanced health care system that has been perpetrated in this country is that people have been educated to believe that the way to cure a disease is to find the one thing that kills off or gets rid of the disease, somehow, the "silver bullet" that specifically targets what is wrong with them.

Unfortunately, a person who is ill is not ill because he has one thing wrong with him, one vitamin missing from his diet, or one disease organism that somehow got loose in his system. He is ill because the body is out of *balance,* and it must be badly out of balance before he gets sick. The body is a homeostatic mechanism (*homeo* = self; *status* = stabilizing), meaning it is cleverly designed to bring itself back to a stable condition in spite of outside influences if it has the necessary ingredients to work with. This is why the body always has a constant temperature, whether we are playing in the snow or sitting in a warm room, unless we are sick—in which case, our fever is an expression of a balanced system working in a natural way to rid the body of an invading foreign organism.

However, the theory of using a chemical to kill disease is what gave rise to the popular habit of taking aspirin when you have a fever. The thought seems to be that if the fever is gone, then the disease must be gone. Quite the contrary—aspirin merely suppresses the symptoms of disease and actually prevents the body from total healing. When drugs are taken over a long period of time, they suppress the symptoms of disease, and toxic residue from infection

26

builds up in the body, which eventually wears down the body and allows chronic diseases to take over.

For example, the chronic aspirin user (to handle headaches or fevers) becomes the ulcer victim later in life. The person who uses antibiotics and cold remedies for colds and the flu retains the toxins from these infections and later experiences other types of inflammatory reactions such as arthritis.

The reason drugs don't work is simple and basic, but it's actually hard to understand because we have been given conflicting data for many years. The use of pharmaceutical drugs does not work because they are based on the primary fallacy of allopathic medicine: "force handles force."

For example, if you have a bacterium that is creating an illness in the body, then you put in something that will kill this bacterium, and this is supposed to handle the disease. In other words, there is a force creating an undesirable situation in the body (the bacterium), so we put in another force to counteract the force of the bacterium, and assume the body is going to get well. Obviously, this is a principle around which many people in Western societies base their lives, so it is not surprising that this philosophy would be prevalent in Western "scientific" medicine.

However, the truth of the matter is that force *never* handles force. You could look at any example in the society around you, and you will see this is true. War is the most striking example, obviously. It is a force designed to counteract the force that some neighboring society is putting up against another. If you look at history textbooks, you will understand that war never resolves anything; war always leads to a situation that creates another war. I am not a pacifist, and I am not arguing for pacifism here. I am just stating a principle on which life operates.

This is simply to show you that one underlying principle of life is that using force against force does not produce positive results; however, other elements can be brought in to resolve a situation in which two forces are opposing each other, thereby creating a more optimum situation.

Let's look an example in the body. An individual has a fever of 103° caused by a viral infection. The simple way of resolving this with force would be to assume the body is too hot. Then, once we have identified the problem, we would say, "Let's cool it off." If force worked against force, we would put the person in a cold bath, chill the body to a more optimum temperature, and this would get rid of the illness. Well, you say, that example is absurd, and, of course, it is. Yet it is an example of attempting to use force to resolve a situation in the body in which there is less than optimal force acting upon the body, *i.e.,* the illness.

Nutrition operates on quite a different set of principles. Regaining health through nutrition operates by ameliorating a troubling condition in the body by providing the body with the correct nutrients necessary to resolve the conflict, rather than fight harder against the opposing force.

Homeopathy employs an even more sophisticated method of resolving unwanted force in the body. This type of treatment actually creates a situation in the body in which there is a miniature duplication of the imbalance. This enables the body to get rid of the unwanted force by matching the electromagnetic make-up of the illness.

The guiding principle and belief of nutritionists is that no drug, vitamin, or other chemical can cure the body; nor, for that matter, does any doctor or nutritionist. The body *cures itself*, given the opportunity and the nutrients it needs.

The only way we can work to truly cure disease is to rid the body's environment of chemicals and other pollutants that prevent it from curing itself, and then give it the necessary nutrients to do so. This is the only way, and it is also a universally successful way. When I have worked with someone in this manner, they have not only freed themselves of the particular malady they were suffering from, but they also become healthier and more energetic.

Sadly, the nutritionist usually has little opportunity to do something this simple with his or her clients. In my experience, the majority of people take the path of least resistance in trying to handle an unwanted physical condition. They go along with the cultural acceptance of drugs, radiation, and surgery to try to handle the problem, until they find out years later that they have created wreckage in their bodies. *Then*, after years of symptom suppression, they realize there has to be a better way, and they come seeking the advice of the nutritionist.

In this case, the nutritionist not only has to work against the damage the disease and drugs have done to the body, but also against the lies that the medical system has fed the person along with the drugs.

I once had a lady come to me who had suffered a stroke and was being given Coumadin by her doctor to prevent further blood clots. She wanted to get healthy. But her doctor told her she must be on Coumadin the rest of her life, a statement she accepted as truth. Now, Coumadin is identical to warfarin, a widely used rat poison. It causes the blood to become thin and prevents clotting. This is how it kills rats; they bleed to death internally. Suppose I had put this lady on a diet and nutritional supplements to bring her body back into balance. Her blood would have been brought back to normal—in which case she might have suffered a hemorrhage in the brain that would have killed her, due to the fact that she also had "rat poison" circulating in her system. Yet, she somehow expected me to make her healthy at the same time she was taking the poison given to her by her doctor!

Obviously, I could not accept her as a client. Nutritionists are legally prevented from telling a person to stop taking pharmaceutical medications, because this is considered "prescribing." In my experience as a nutritionist, I can only help my client achieve optimum results if the client tells me that he wants to get off medical drugs, and intends to do so gradually as he becomes healthier.

In the view of a nutritionist, obviously, nutrition should be tried *first* in the presence of illness. Once a person has experienced the full devastation of drugs, radiation, and surgery, it becomes more difficult to overcome disease with more natural methods.

3

Your Body and It's Environment

nce upon a time, there was a Garden of Eden. The climate was perfect, so no one had to wear man-made synthetic fabrics for clothing or burn fossil fuels to keep warm. There was no electromagnetic pollution from power lines, TVs, nuclear fallout, or other forms of radiation. All of the food was organically grown and could be plucked from trees; it was quite plentiful. In this kind of situation, the body functioned perfectly and did not encounter any diseases that it was not fully equipped to handle.

Well, maybe or maybe not. At any rate, our bodies are related to animal bodies in their functioning, whether you consider that we evolved from "lower forms of life" or not. As with other animals, our bodies were originally designed to eat the foodstuffs that naturally occur on this planet. Primitive people did not need to be equipped with lead shields to ward off nuclear fallout, microwave radiation, or other forms of radiant pollution. Likewise, they did not need extensive filtration systems to clean the air of smog and other contaminants they might breathe in, because the air was naturally clean.

Human bodies are not well equipped to survive in our present-day environment. This is obvious when we look at all the animal species that have gone extinct over the last hundred years as a result of man's actions. The only question that remains is: Have we fouled our own nest to the extent that we will also go the way of the California condor, the snail darter, and the dinosaur?

Now, we are not just considering obvious pollution here. Most of us are aware of the fact that we live in a fairly heavily polluted environment. But we often feel that if we eat "health foods," we can counteract the effects of our environment to some degree. What we call "good" food, however, is not necessarily what the human body was designed to eat.

One of the most obvious differences between the present human diet and that of other animals is that we cook our food. I'm not saying we should go back to eating raw foods, because I believe humans have lived on cooked foods for so long that the human body has adapted to some extent to these foods. In addition, we do not do well on a completely raw food diet, although some nutritionists might disagree with me on this point!

Something that passes most people's attention, however, is the fact that most of the food that we consider "natural" has been intensively bred away from being a natural wild food in order to produce more "desirable" traits. These traits include more tenderness, *i.e.,* more water retention, milder flavor, and a lack of certain irritating substances that may be present in the wild predecessor. This often means they have also been bred to contain less of the nutrients the body needs. For example, in Ewell Gibbons' book *Stalking the Wild Asparagus* he mentions some analyses that he had done on certain wild greens, which he found many, many times higher in Vitamins A and C than the greens we normally grow in our gardens and consider quite nourishing. It is widely known that the wheat now being produced in the United States has a much lower concentration of protein than wheat grown in the same areas 50 or 100 years ago. This could be partially due to the depletion of the soil, but it could also be due to the fact that wheat strains have been bred selectively to produce a higher yield per acre, without measuring whether this yield was in terms of starch or in terms of protein. I'm not saying that we should all go back to browsing in the forest, but I do want to point out the problem with our food and the environment in which we find ourselves.

Many people have complained to me that they don't want to take vitamin pills for the rest of their lives. They want to get all the nutrients they need from natural foods. But, as I have pointed out, it can be quite difficult to find anything that qualifies as a totally "natural" food.

So what are we to do with a body that was designed for a "Garden of Eden," now that we are bombarded with toxic chemicals we have no mechanisms for handling, and we are being fed foods that simply do not have the necessary nutrients to combat our polluted environment? Fortunately, there are some steps we can take to create a situation more to the body's liking.

If we analyze and lay out a program for creating an ideal environment for our bodies, it would probably include the following:

1. Avoid air pollution as much as possible. If you must live in the city because it's a more profitable environment for your work, then for goodness sake you'd better make enough money to equip your house and your car with devices that precipitate out some of the more toxic airborne pollutants. This would include an air filtration system for the house and negative ion generators for the house and the car.

2. Purchase good water. It's an added expense, but even the best tap water is contaminated these days. The very best water is mountain water that comes from glacier-fed springs. This water is high in minerals that are not dissolved, but are in colloidal suspension. This is the best way for the body to accept minerals. Please see Chapter 7 "The Value of Pure Water" for more information.

3. Eat the highest quality foods available. Foods grown on highly mineralized soil, with a heavy addition of organic material

(natural fertilizers), and that is certified pesticide-free is the best food you can get in our present environment. It can be difficult to find quality fruits and vegetables unless you grow your own, but farmers' markets can be a good source of organic produce.

4. Eat as much raw food as you find comfortable in your diet. In addition, you will likely need to rely on natural nutritional supplements, not necessarily "vitamins." In fact, high doses of vitamins and minerals can often be quite toxic, and I certainly do not recommend that anyone self-dose with megavitamins, as they can do long-term damage. Natural whole-food concentrates are preferable, such as some herbal foods and those made by Standard Process Labs.

5. Get as much exercise as possible in an environment that is as free of pollution as possible. If you are a runner, that's great. But for heaven's sake, don't go out and run on the city streets choked with vehicle exhaust at 5:00 p.m. This will simply exchange the carbon dioxide in your lungs for lead and other pollutants. Many gyms and spas are oblivious to this problem, and they often use all sorts of cleaning solvents that leave toxic vapors in the air. So just be aware of this, and choose your exercise environment as best you can.

There really is no Garden of Eden left on this planet, because pollution has become so global there isn't anywhere we can "escape to." So, in addition to the five steps above, I would recommend another important step:

6. Take responsibility for your environment. Recognize the sources of pollution and do what you can to eliminate them. Yes, recycling the tin cans, the glass, and the newspapers helps to some extent, but I don't think that's going to save us. We must educate ourselves and follow the steps given above as much as possible. We must also educate our government and

the people who run the companies that make the products the public demands, but that also contribute to the desecration of the environment on this planet. You can do a lot as an individual to help reverse this situation. Thank you for doing as much as you can to create a more perfect and healthy environment!

4

How the
Body Heals

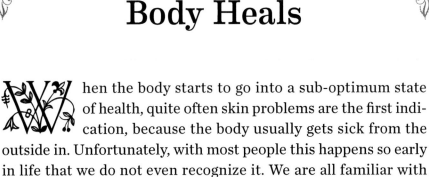

hen the body starts to go into a sub-optimum state of health, quite often skin problems are the first indication, because the body usually gets sick from the outside in. Unfortunately, with most people this happens so early in life that we do not even recognize it. We are all familiar with babies getting diaper rash and other skin rashes, and they "grow out of it," which actually means their symptoms progress to a deeper layer of the body.

As teenagers, most people experience pimples, which are signs of the body's attempt to get rid of toxins. Usually, pimples are suppressed by some kind of acne cream, or worse, antibiotics, and again the teenager "grows out of it." However, with this type of symptom suppression, the disease will progress into deeper layers. We are not talking about particular diseases, but the general state of health as the body regresses from normal to subnormal.

The body heals from the inside out. The last indicator that a person is getting well is usually a skin problem, which makes it seem like the person's health is getting worse. This is sometimes referred to as a "detox reaction" or "healing crisis." This state of progression often occurs when someone begins eating natural foods and other nutrients to gradually improve their health.

There is another type of progression of healing we need to look at in order understand some of the phenomena that occur during the healing process.

When one organ or a portion of the body is diseased, we could say it has been selected as a repository for disease. This part of the body will tend to go out of communication with the rest of the body. The nerve supply to this particular portion is reduced, the circulation is reduced, and that portion of the body may actually be "walled off" by a layer of antibodies that surrounds the tissue. The area becomes numb, and the person usually has little awareness of it after it has been diseased for some time, because communication with the troubled area is poor.

Let's look at an example. Suppose there is a fungal infection in the spleen. The toxins produced in the spleen due to the infection will cause an irritation of the nerves leading to that area, and this can actually react back along the nerves that innervate the spleen from the spinal cord. This can cause a partial shutting down of the nerve supply from the spinal cord. Many chiropractors will tell you that it doesn't matter which comes first, a *subluxation*—a slight misalignment of the vertebrae leading to pinching of the nerve that runs between them—or the disease, because either one will react back to the other end of the communication line and affect the other one. As a result of this lack of enervation, circulation to the organ shuts down to a certain extent, which means the organ will receive a lesser supply of nutrients and waste products will accumulate, rather than being eliminated. The infected spleen now becomes a diseased area resembling a foreign invading organism. Therefore, the body produces antibodies to it and actually walls it off.

Thus, we now have a condition in which the spleen is very much out of communication with the rest of the body. So what happens when we start healing it? First of all, if we were to do a chiropractic adjustment in the area of the back containing the nerve to the spleen area, we would find that area of the back is out of alignment. An adjustment to this area would increase the nerve flow. This, in turn, would increase circulation to the spleen. So now we have a chance for the organ to come into better communication with the rest of the body.

However, the spleen will then start dumping toxins, creating a backlash along the communication line. This, in turn, creates more irritation in the nerve, usually resulting in the vertebrae (which has just been adjusted) going back out of alignment. Thus, one can go back many, many times to a chiropractor for the same adjustment, only to find that it must be done over and over again. Hopefully, after a long period of time, balance can be restored and the adjustment will start to hold.

In addition, the toxins now being released into the surrounding tissues are likely to cause inflammation around the spleen because we have released poisons into them, and these poisons must be removed. The way the body does this is to increase the temperature and circulation in the affected area, resulting in redness and inflammation.

One of the things that health professionals can use in treating a diseased organ is an extract of that organ from another animal. It might simply be desiccated tissue, or it may be what is called *protomorphogen extract* (an extract that concentrates the genetic material). This type of extract helps repair the communication of the affected organ with its own cells. If you think back to the statement above that the body has built an antibody layer around the diseased organ, the spleen in this example, then you can understand what will happen when we add either desiccated spleen or spleen protomorphogen to the diet of the afflicted individual. The spleen tissue we put in will react with the antibodies because they are antibodies to spleen. Therefore, the person may well experience more pain in the area because these antibodies are being precipitated. However, this reaction is essential because the antibodies make up the wall that the body uses to cut the communication with the spleen. Therefore, one of the purposes of giving a person spleen extract is to precipitate out the antibodies and allow the spleen to get back in communication with the rest of the body. This is the theory behind the products developed by Standard Process Labs.

In my experience, a program of chiropractic and good nutrition can start the total healing process in the body, along with taking tissue extract of the particular organ that is most affected by disease.

Now let's take a look at an example in which we *don't* do this. Let's say a person comes in with a diseased spleen, but this is not his primary complaint. Indeed, he's not aware that his spleen is diseased because it has been out of communication with the rest of the body for so long that he no longer has awareness of it. Let's say he complains about skin rashes. Now, we can put him on an intense program to handle skin rashes, and when we do this the body starts to get better. Now, the body has already gone out of communication with the spleen because the spleen was in a much worse condition than the rest of the body. If you can imagine a picture of the body rising up to a higher condition of health, and the spleen not getting healthier, then you can see we are actually creating a dangerous situation in which the condition of the spleen can get worse.

This is why it has been so difficult for health professionals to treat people with nutrition in order to bring them back to health. It is not obvious from the symptoms that an individual reports, and sometimes not even from medical tests, that there is a diseased and isolated portion of the body.

Schools of healing with long histories of practice, such as clinical herbology (healing with herbs) homeopathy, and chiropractic have developed systems of getting around the problem of communication with the body. Applied Kinesiology and similar techniques offer an excellent way to communicate directly with the body concerning what it needs to come back into balance, including its nutritional needs.

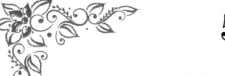

5

Diet for Optimum Health

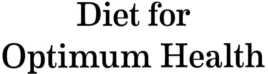

umans evolve. Thus, we have people with dark brown skin living near the equator and blue-eyed blondes living in northern Europe. The evolutionary reason for this is that dark skin filters out the damaging rays of the sun, which adds to survival levels in areas with intense sunlight; whereas, pale skin allows the body surface to get more sunlight with which to produce Vitamin D.

So why should we expect one diet to be best for everyone? Many nutritionists have made this mistake, often by studying some particularly healthy group of people and then pronouncing that the whole world should eat the same diet.

This gives rise to such atrocious situations as well-intentioned public health workers trying to get African-American children to drink more milk. The truth of the matter is that these children's African ancestors never saw a cow, never tasted milk other than that of their mothers, and lost the enzymes to digest it quite early in life. As a result, there are whole groups of African-Americans growing up with chronic diarrhea and never understanding why, unless they just happen to stop drinking milk.

No, a diet must be tailored to the individual. Fortunately, nature provides a method for doing this—we have taste buds—and they are fairly well tuned to appreciate the foods we most require in our diet, *providing* we have only natural foods to choose from.

But there's the problem. The entire food processing industry in America is geared towards fooling our taste buds. This is the sum total of billions of dollars' worth of business—to convince our taste buds to accept something that makes the industry a large profit, but that is of little value to the body. So the obvious conclusion is that we need to get highly processed foods out of our diets. Once we do this, our natural ability to choose food according to what our bodies need begins to assert itself..

Of course, food is an emotional subject, and it often takes some time of living on a whole-food diet for the concept that love is equal to ice cream and Grandma's chocolate chip cookies to die away. Once we get to this point, we can approach diet in a more rational way.

Dr. Huntley's Dietary Guidelines

Your diet should be high in complex carbohydrates, because they are digested slowly and feed the body for a long period of time after eating. The nutrients in the food are gradually released into the bloodstream. Usually, this is in the form of grains. Most root vegetable carbohydrates, such as potatoes and carrots, are more rapidly digested and can end up being stored in the form of fat.

WHOLE GRAINS

Grains are an important staple food for the human body. They have been found in most cultures for, perhaps, millions of years. In the United States, grains have been almost totally eliminated from the diet except in the form of flours, usually wheat, which are often bleached and usually degermed—meaning the most nourishing part of the grain has been removed. This provides us with a pasty substance that does offer some calories and which—for the benefit of the food industry—lasts a long time on the shelf. Whole grain is another matter.

Whole grain is seed from a grass that has been harvested and usually the outer layer, the husk, has been removed. Whole grain can be cooked as is, or it can be ground coarsely to make meal or finely to make flour. Whole grains are a source of a great deal of nutrition. Not only do they provide complex carbohydrates in the form of starch that nourish the body slowly without putting a stress on the sugar-handling mechanisms, they also contains significant amounts of protein, minerals, certain essential vitamins, and some essential fatty acids in their natural form.

The best way to preserve nutrients is to keep the whole grain kernel intact. Therefore, flour is the worst alternative we have for eating grain. When you make grain into flour, it has to be ground quite finely, and many of its surfaces are exposed to oxygen, which destroys many of the nutrients in the grain.

Ideally, there are two ways to eat grain:

1. Sprouted, in which case the whole kernel is soaked in water long enough for it to swell and take up enough water to start it growing. It is then allowed to sprout for a day or more, which changes it into a growing food that is more like a vegetable than a seed. Most grains are not eaten this way, although commonly other beans and seeds are; the most widely used are alfalfa and mung beans.

2. The most common way to eat grains is to cook them whole. Once cooked, they can be added to other foods, including soups and stews, or used to make breads and other baked foods.

In selecting grains, it again becomes important to select fresh grains. However, the freshness of grain is not quite as obvious as it is with fresh fruits and vegetables. I have had people come to me and say they bought grain at a widely known chain of "health food stores," and they did not know what to do with it when they got home because there were little bugs crawling around in it. Well, at this point, it becomes obvious that your grain is quite stale, indeed! Hopefully, you will never have this experience. However, any sign of excessive dust, cobweb-like material, or mold on grain is a clear sign it is stale and should not be used.

Your best bet in attempting to find fresh whole grains is to buy them from a reliable source. After you have experienced the taste of grain that is very, very fresh, and that has been stored properly so as to maintain the freshness, compared to the rather stale grains that we often find at grocery stores, you will never settle for second best again.

The most stabilizing grain for most people is barley, preferably in the form of whole, pearled barley. Also important is brown rice. All grains should be eaten whole. Flour products, including bread, do not promote health. The greater your desire for improved health, the higher the percentage of whole grains should be in your diet, up to 60 percent of your diet. If you are in good health, you can have whole grain breads (preferably sprouted) and whole grain noodles in addition to actual whole grains.

Other grains that may be of benefit to some people are millet, buckwheat (primarily for winter use), rye, teff, and quinoa. Wheat causes reactions in many people, so it should be avoided unless you have been specifically tested for it. Oats, oatmeal, and dried corn products, such as cornmeal and popcorn, also do not promote health in most people. These grains generally promote the growth of fungi.

For maximum health improvement, eat at least one large serving of barley and one of brown rice each day. See "Dr. Huntley's Foolproof Recipe for Delicious Brown Rice" in Part II.

Different people might need different types of grain. Northern climates grow wheat and buckwheat well. People of northern European descent do well on these grains *provided* they live in a cool climate. These grains contain gluten. Gluten is not found in a high concentration in rice, barley, and millet, which are staples for people living nearer the equator. Gluten is not well tolerated by descendants of these people. Here, again, we find the health of African-Americans being affected by a diet of wheat ("white") bread being forced on them.

While we can't "adapt" our ancestors, we can adapt our diet to the kind of climate we live in. People who live in a warm climate will find their bodies feeling overheated easily if they eat wheat and buckwheat frequently. They would do better on rice, millet, and barley. But the tradition of buckwheat pancakes to warm you up on a frosty morning is quite valid.

Now, grains are not a complete diet. If they are grown on good soil, they contain considerable protein, but it is not complete protein. This means the amino acids in the protein are not in exactly the right balance to enable the body to build new tissue.

Therefore, grains need balancing proteins in the form of small amounts of beans, fish, meat, or other high-protein foods to complement the amino acids in the grain. But the amount of these necessary heavier proteins is quite small in comparison to the conventional American idea regarding how much meat we should eat. In a warm climate, perhaps the average person needs two ounces a day. In a cold climate, he may need more because the body tends to burn it up for fuel rapidly. Thus, we have Eskimos, who are quite healthy on a diet of largely meat and fat, a diet that would rapidly kill someone living in Southern California.

VEGETABLES

Your diet should contain large amounts of vegetables. Vegetables contain vitamins and minerals essential for the body's maintenance, without which it cannot function. They also contain bulk, which helps normalize the intestinal flora and prevent toxins from building up in the system. The vegetables should include both non-starchy root vegetables (carrots, daikon radish, turnips, onion, garlic, rutabagas, parsnips, and more) and greens (cabbage, kale, dark green lettuce, and sprouts of all kinds), with small amounts of other vegetables (squash, tomatoes, cucumbers, peppers, and more). Starchy root vegetables, such as potatoes, should only be eaten occasionally, because the starch they contain is more rapidly digested than that found in grains. Therefore, they contribute to obesity.

Vegetables in the nightshade family: white potatoes, tomatoes, bell peppers, and eggplant, should be avoided or eaten in limited amounts. These vegetables contain a toxin that is difficult for the body to handle, and they can cause joint pain, including rheumatoid arthritis and other problems. Tomatoes should be eaten with meat.

Most vegetables are best digested if they are lightly cooked. Winter squashes and other hard vegetables should be cooked until tender. They can be steamed, baked, or stir-fried (at low temperature with little oil). If water is used in cooking vegetables, the water should always be used (with the vegetables or in soups) because many of the nutrients in the vegetables dissolve in water.

In warm weather, you may also enjoy greens and other vegetables as salads. Do not use vinegar or bottled dressings on your salad. The best dressing is one made of olive oil and lemon juice, with seasonings added.

FRUIT

Fruit is a valuable food that contains essential vitamins and minerals, plus it cleans the digestive tract. However, fruit contains sugar, so be careful with it. If you are having problems with Candida, diabetes, or low blood sugar, it is best to avoid fruit. If you have fruit in your diet, eat it only as your first food in the morning, and then 1 to 2 pieces at bedtime, if desired. Do not eat fruit with meals, as it prevents proper digestion of other foods. Do not eat dried fruit, because it is a concentrated sweet. Fruit juices should be avoided at the beginning of your cleansing program. If you are attempting to gain weight, on the other hand, then fruit should be eaten ½ to 1 hour before a meal in order to stimulate the appetite.

Fruit eaten with other foods (especially high-protein foods) inhibits digestion because the fruit sugar is digested and absorbed quite rapidly. Proteins, which take some time to digest, often are not completely digested if eaten with fruit. This can lead to intestinal gas, stomach upset, and possibly more serious problems.

FERMENTED FOODS

Traditional diets in most cultures contain some kind of fermented foods. These are quite important in maintaining a balanced intestinal flora. Whether it be yogurt, kefir, true sauerkraut (not the artificial kind made with vinegar), miso, poi, or umeboshi plums, it is important that some fermented food be eaten every day to aid in digestion of the other food you eat. Sorry, beer doesn't count, because the yeast used in making the beer produces alcohol, not the lactic acid that keeps the intestines healthy!

SEAWEED

Seaweeds contain valuable trace minerals (including iodine) rarely found in other foods. Wakame, hiziki, and nori are excellent. Only a small amount (1 teaspoon to 1 tablespoon) of dried seaweed needs to be eaten daily to supplement the diet. This may be cooked in soups and added to other vegetables.

In areas where the food is grown in rich soils that have not been depleted by the use of soluble fertilizers, then vegetables and grains grown on these soils are adequate. Such areas rarely exist in the United States, however, so I recommend a small amount of seaweed of some sort in the diet daily. It also helps to eat fish frequently as a protein source.

CONDIMENTS

These are essential to most people's enjoyment of their food. However, excessive use of strong condiments such as salt, vinegar, and pepper, can be quite irritating and unbalancing to the body, as can sauces that combine fat and starch.

SALT

Salt is so overused in our society that natural foods taste quite flat to people who are used to a fast-food lifestyle. Often, this can be remedied by using sesame salt, a mixture of one part sea salt to 15 parts roasted sesame seeds. The salt and sesame seeds are ground together and provide a delicious condiment that tastes much more "salty" than it actually is. This traditional Japanese condiment should be ground in a suribachi bowl (available in Japanese groceries or some health food stores) to give the right mixture of whole and ground seeds. This is a delicious salt, but it can go rancid rapidly, so you will need to store it in a cool, dark place in order for it to remain tasty and healthful. If you refrigerate it, you must seal it and then let it come to room temperature before you unwrap it, or it will pick up a lot of moisture.

CAUTION: If you have high blood pressure, be sure to limit your intake of tamari (soy sauce) and miso, as these fermented products contain a large amount of salt.

FATS AND OILS

High quality oils are essential in your diet to produce good health. Essential fatty acids are found in unrefined oils and are used by your body to make cell membranes, which are extremely important in healing. The best oil for repairing the body is unrefined flax oil made using a special process that was developed by Dr. Johanna Budwig in Germany. Dr. Budwig is known for developing a cure for cancer and chronic diseases using organic flaxseed oil combined with organic low-fat cottage cheese. This specific dietary protocol is called "The Budwig Diet." (See References.)

Cold-pressed, organic flaxseed oil can be added to cold foods, such as salads. For cooking and seasoning, use fresh raw or organic butter, olive oil, sesame, canola, or other unrefined oils. Always keep oil in the refrigerator, even olive oil, although you may have to take it out for a few minutes before using to warm it up enough to pour. Oil that is left warm goes rancid and is harmful to your health.

Foods that contain high amounts of oil, such as avocados, almonds, sesame seeds, and wheat germ, may be valuable additions to your diet, but only if they are quite fresh. Make certain they are fresh when you buy them, and refrigerate or freeze them when you get home.

Do not fry or deep fry food. Occasionally, you can have foods that are stir-fried; this means they are, heated in a small amount of oil for a short time to improve their flavor. Coconut oil is the best oil for this type of cooking, because it does not break down quickly when heated. You can cook delicious vegetables by stir-frying them in oil for a minute and then adding a few spoonfuls of water. Cover the pot tightly and let the vegetables steam in this water-oil mixture until just barely tender. Do not drain off the liquid, but use it as a natural sauce to serve with vegetables.

Avoid margarine. It's a synthetic food that cannot build health, in spite of the claims made for its value.

How do you tell if fats or oils are rancid? Develop a good sense of smell! If you take a fresh stick of butter and smell it, you will discover it has a pleasing odor. Nuts that have been recently picked from the tree and cracked open and eaten immediately will have a pleasant fragrance. These are fresh oils. Now, take a package of roasted nuts that have been roasted in oil, and leave some of the nuts out on the counter for several weeks. Notice the change in odor. The oil has become rancid. You must develop your sense of taste and odor, because this will allow you to distinguish between fresh and stale or rancid food. Unfortunately, it is quite common—almost the rule—for rancid oils to be found in our food. Most of the oils available in the marketplace have had most of the essential fatty acids removed in order to make them more stable.

Recent technology has brought to light that only oils extracted by pressing in refrigerated environments in the dark and in an oxygen-free atmosphere truly retain the essential fatty acids. This means that most of the foods that we have relied on as a source of fat in our diet are severely inadequate. Even so-called "cold pressed" oils actually are normally pressed in a screw press, which generates a considerable amount of heat, thus damaging the oil. At the same time, they are exposed to light and oxygen, and much of the essential fatty acid content is destroyed. There are some new products on the market that are produced in a cold, dark, and oxygen-free environment. These are the only oils that should be used to any extent in the diet, and, of course, they cannot be used for cooking because they will go rancid quite rapidly when subjected to heat.

When looking at the use of oils in the diet, we see that the most critical factor is the ratio of essential fatty acid to oil, because all fats and oils require essential fatty acids in their digestion. Therefore, it is wise to restrict your use of fat unless your diet is supplemented with essential fatty acid-rich oil.

Spectrum Naturals and Arrowhead Mills make such oils. Pressed Veg-Omega-3 certified organic fresh Flax Oil is often used as a nutritional supplement. This oil is so rich in essential fatty acids that it must never be heated. It must be kept refrigerated until immediately before eating.

The most important thing to remember when you are planning a diet to improve your health is that all foods should be fresh. Never eat stale or rancid foods, or any foods that have been on the shelf too long. Your body needs fresh, whole foods that contain all their natural nutritional elements to build optimum health. For this reason, you should avoid canned, frozen, or otherwise preserved foods.

DESSERTS

Desserts and sweeteners should generally be avoided, although some people can have maple syrup, brown rice syrup, or barley malt syrup. Check with your nutritional consultant as to whether you would benefit from one of these sweeteners. Desserts should be made of whole grains or whole-grain flours, and sweetened only with rice syrup, barley malt, or a small amount of cooked fruits. Rice syrup and barley malt are complex carbohydrates that taste sweet, but they don't produce the effect of releasing sugar into the bloodstream as rapidly as other sweeteners do. Cooked fruit doesn't have the enzymes that raw fruit does, and it does not create the fermentation in the stomach that causes indigestion due to combining fresh fruit with proteins. Maple syrup is a concentrated sweetener that can be used in dessert recipes instead of cane sugar. It actually has the beneficial property of killing some of the harmful fungi in the intestines, but it may be too sweet for some people at some point in their nutritional healing program.

General Guidelines

The following general guidelines are intended to help you start cleansing your body and transition into a diet that suits the overall state of your metabolism.

These foods should be eliminated:

- All milk products, except plain yogurt, kefir, Camembert or Brie cheese (limit to 4 ounces per week) and raw butter
- All sweets, except those made with barley malt syrup or rice syrup
- Fried foods, except foods that are stir-fried with a tiny amount of cold-pressed unrefined oil
- Bread, except Ezekiel or Essene

- Carbonated beverages
- Iced drinks, which are hard on the kidneys
- Alcoholic drinks of any kind. In a few months, you can try natural beers. Make sure you have been tested to see if you need specific treatment for *Candida albicans* (overgrowth of fungus, usually found in the digestive tract) before you even consider adding anything that contains alcohol to your diet.
- Prepared salad dressings
- Heavily spiced foods
- All food additives, preservatives, artificial sweeteners, and other chemicals in food. In general, avoid prepackaged, canned, and frozen foods. No hydrogenated fats, often found in store-bought baked goods.

These foods should be limited:
- Red meat once a week. People with type O blood must be cautious when consuming red meat.
- Coffee, tea, and other drinks with caffeine as much as possible
- Fresh fruit, only first thing in the morning. Some people can eat fruit between meals, but do not eat fruit with meals.

Dietary Schedule

Upon arising:
- Taking supplements on an empty stomach is recommended; take them when you get up and wait ½ hour before eating fruit.
- Eat as much fruit and/or juice (preferably fresh) as desired.
- Exercise outdoors for 20 minutes, if possible.

Then eat breakfast:
- Scrambled tofu (with or without added steamed vegetables), or,

- 1 to 2 eggs with Ezekiel toast (small amount of raw butter if desired) OR whole-grain cereal with almond milk

Lunch and Dinner:

- Two servings of vegetables
- Steamed, baked, or stir-fried seafood, fish, tofu, or chicken (red meat occasionally)
- Whole grains
- Salad if desired (no iceberg lettuce; use greens or sprouts)
- Use tomatoes only if meat is also eaten.
- Drink as little as possible with the meal. If you are thirsty, drink as much water as desired before you sit down to eat.

Recommended seasonings:

- Miso in sauce or soup
- Sesame salt
- All herbs
- Tamari or other fermented soy sauce
- Lemon juice
- Umeboshi plum paste
- Raw butter in small amounts

More About Foods to Avoid!

Most people should avoid milk products, including milk, cheese, buttermilk, and cream. They produce excessive mucus in the body. When your body is cleaning out toxins, you are likely to be more uncomfortable if you include milk or milk products in your diet. People who are in good health may have small amounts of well-fermented cheeses, such as Brie and Camembert. Some people find that yogurt and kefir do not create mucus, but check with your nutritional consultant before you add these to your diet. Raw butter is okay because it does not contain mucus-producing milk protein.

Carbonated beverages, including mineral waters, often disrupt proper digestion of food. Iced drinks can also disrupt digestion. Digestive enzymes in your stomach cannot work if your stomach is chilled. These enzymes also do not work properly when diluted, so avoid drinking any more liquid than necessary with your meals. Avoid alcohol of any kind. It is a poison. You are trying to build health, not death! Avoid coffee, black tea, and any other sources of caffeine. Caffeine is an addictive drug and does not belong in a healing program. In addition, coffee and many dark teas contain toxins that promote the growth of fungi. Some herbal teas are okay, but check with your nutritional consultant for the specific ones allowed in your diet.

Tobacco is an addictive drug that has quite damaging effects on the body. Your body cannot repair itself when you are taking in something that is so destructive.

Avoid canned foods, food additives, preservatives, and any other foods you know or suspect contain chemicals. To build health, your body needs natural foods, not artificially produced additives.

You should also avoid the harmful chemicals that are found in the products you use on the outside of your body, because they can be absorbed through the skin. This means you should not use deodorants containing aluminum, mineral oil as a body lotion, or other toxic lotions or perfumes. Do not use toothpaste that contains fluoride, or shampoo with sodium laurel sulfate. Also, do not cook your food in aluminum pots, because some of the aluminum is leached into the food. Use stainless steel, enamel, glass, or crockery.

Food Combining

Food combining is a controversial subject, and with good reason. It is an individually variable subject, meaning certain "rules" of food combining apply to certain people and not to others.

People who believe intensely in food combining will tell you that proteins should not be eaten with starches under any conditions. On the other hand, there are those who cheerfully combine these for dinner every day of their lives with no ill effects that they are aware of.

Just as some people have a lighter metabolism than others, meaning they cannot eat lots of carbohydrates and meats, whereas others can, so also do some people have a digestive tract that is sensitive to particular combinations of food that other people can digest easily. So, let us deal with some of the most obvious examples of food combining here, and then indicate that the rest is up to your particular sensitivity and your discretion.

It is difficult to combine melon with other foods. No one seems to be quite aware of the reason for this, but it has been a fairly obvious observation of those who have studied food combinations for years. Melon in itself is not easy for a lot of people to digest, and so the food-combining rule that seems best is: Always eat melon alone, or leave it alone.

Another fairly obvious rule of food combining is in the combination of fresh fruits with other foods. Fresh foods have their own enzymes and undergo their own digestive process in the stomach. This is quite a rapid process, in which the food is broken down easily and the sugar is released rapidly into the bloodstream directly from the stomach. When fruit is eaten with other cooked foods (particularly protein) the release of sugar into the bloodstream signals the body that digestion in the stomach is complete, and the contents of the stomach are then emptied rapidly into the small intestine. As a result, the protein that was eaten is passed along not completely digested, giving rise to lower bowel gas and much intestinal discomfort later in the digestive process. A safe rule to follow is simply: Do not eat fresh fruit with complete meals; eat it alone.

The emphasis on eating lots of fresh food in recent years has led a number of people to make the uncomfortable mistake of believing that for good health they should have fresh fruit for dessert rather than cooked dessert. This attempt at a healthy diet leads to great intestinal distress, and these people (if they are lucky) arrives at the nutritionist's office thinking that in spite of the attempts to get healthier they are feeling worse. Educating people about not eating fresh fruit during the day often clears this up.

With the majority of people, this actually extends so far as to say that they should not eat fresh fruit anytime during the day, assuming they have consumed an adequate (for them) amount of fresh fruit in the early morning. They should refrain from eating fresh fruit simply because of the changes it creates in the blood sugar, which, in turn, interferes with the digestive process.

Protein-starch combinations are much more controversial because some people seem to do quite well on some of these combinations. In particular, the traditional oriental combination of brown rice and fish seems to be an easily digested combination for many people.

The American "ideal meal" of steak and baked potato can be disastrous for the digestive tract. Most people assimilate potato starch quite rapidly. This starch acts much like a sugar, but steak needs a long time in the stomach. So, many people get the same problem with this combination as with fresh fruit and a heavy meal. Anyone who is having health (and particularly digestive) problems should try to eat only one food at a time for a while to give their digestion a chance to sort it all out. Then they can try simple combinations to find the optimum food combinations that work for them.

What to Do About Candida Albicans

If you have been diagnosed with the fungus Candida albicans, the following diet should be followed to heal the fungal overgrowth. Your nutritional consultant will tell you how long you should maintain this diet.

These foods are permitted:

- Bread: Essene bread or Manna bread, or other *yeast-free* breads

- Barley: As much as you want

- Rice: (preferably brown) and millet

- 100 percent pure maple syrup. This is actually therapeutic, because pure maple syrup actually kills Candida! This surprise puts an end to terrible sugar cravings while you're working to get rid of Candida.

WARNING: Maple syrup in the grocery store can be labeled as "pure" when it actually contains 50 percent sugar water. Make certain you purchase it from a reputable health food store and check the label.

- Lots of vegetables

- Meat and fish, preferably purchased from a health store that sells meat certified to contain no chemicals, including hormones and antibiotics

- Butter, olive oil

- Lemon juice

- Fermented foods can be eaten by some people, including miso, plain yogurt, and plain kefir

- Dried shiitake mushrooms

These Foods are *Not* Permitted:

- Avoid any foods that contain yeast, sugars, fungi, or fermented ingredients, including:
- Fruit, fruit juices, or fruit-sweetened products
- Pickles
- Vinegar
- Sweets of any kind, except maple syrup
- Mayonnaise
- Regular bread, because it's made with yeast
- Alcoholic beverages (they are by-products of yeast fermentation)
- Mushrooms (they are a fungus)
- Wheat or corn products (except sprouted wheat)
- B Vitamins (usually made from yeast)
- Most milk products (especially cheese)

A large number of people on a Candida program only need to follow this strict diet for a few weeks. If you cheat, it can take months to get rid of Candida. The more completely you avoid the foods that "feed" the fungus, the sooner you will no longer be affected by it.

Fermented foods can be eaten, including miso, plain yogurt, and plain kefir (no sugar), because they produce lactic acid in the intestines that helps combat Candida.

6

On the Subject
of Protein

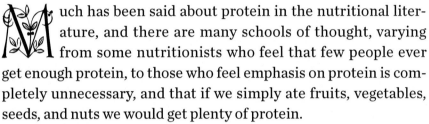uch has been said about protein in the nutritional literature, and there are many schools of thought, varying from some nutritionists who feel that few people ever get enough protein, to those who feel emphasis on protein is completely unnecessary, and that if we simply ate fruits, vegetables, seeds, and nuts we would get plenty of protein.

The truth does not lie somewhere in between, because the truth varies. The optimum amount of protein each individual needs is as different as there are individuals on this planet. It is certainly true that an excess of protein can be quite dangerous to the body. Protein must be broken down and digested, which requires a certain amount of energy. If the protein present in the diet is more than what is required to meet the body's needs for individual amino acids, then the amino acids must be broken down. When this happens, the side group on each amino acid, which contains nitrogen, is broken off of the amino acid and disposed of by converting it into a compound called *urea*, which is then filtered out of the blood by the kidneys and dumped in the form of urine. The rest of the molecule that made up the amino acid is burned for fuel, as is any carbohydrate.

If an excessive amount of amino acids is included in the diet, the kidneys become overworked, and the blood urea content can become high and produce toxic conditions in the body. The breakdown products of nitrogen compounds include ammonia, which is highly toxic, and other hazardous nitrogen-containing compounds.

Once the protein is broken down into amino acids, and the amino acids are further broken down into carbohydrates that can be metabolized, there is no resynthesis of amino acids and the protein is lost to the body.

Basically, this means that eating a large amount of meat, even on rare occasions, overloads the body with toxins without doing a significant amount of good, as far as providing amino acids for protein construction in the body. On the other hand, if inadequate amounts of amino acids are provided in the diet, the body will be deficient in protein, the results of which include muscle wasting, loss of reproduction functions, anemia, and stunted growth in children.

One of the effects of a diet severely deficient in protein is a disease known as *kwashiorkor*, or *edematous malnutrition*, usually seen in African children, who are fed largely on carbohydrates—when there is food, not famine. These children develop stunted growth and bloated stomachs, and they often become mentally retarded due to a severe deficiency of protein. However, it has been shown that less severe forms of protein starvation can also lead to major problems, especially in the area of reproduction. Women who give birth to children during their own growing years, or who live on an extremely protein-deficient diet during their pregnancy, often suffer from major health problems themselves. They are also more likely to give birth to children who have severe problems, including mental retardation.

Unfortunately, it is not just extremely impoverished parents living in other countries who have these problems. In the United States, women often starve themselves, especially those in a profession such as acting or modeling, in order to present a thin, fashionable figure. In so doing, they often become deficient in protein as well as essential fatty acids and other nutrients. It is not infrequent for these women to become infertile and unable to bear children at some point in their lives. We often see protein deficiency in people who live on snack food (or "junk" food) simply because the ratio of non-nutritive carbohydrates to protein is so high that the body is unable to metabolize what little protein is consumed.

The rather obvious solution is to eat foods that have moderate protein content but that do not have an excessive amount of concentrated protein. This includes whole grains, legumes, nuts, and seeds. All of these things are fairly high in protein if they are grown properly, and they can serve as quite adequate protein sources for most people. The need for concentrated protein sources such as meat, eggs, and cheese is minimal, and probably not essential for anyone except people with type O blood. People who are under high stress might require a great deal of protein. This includes athletes, growing children, and pregnant women, who might feel the need to supplement their diet with these animal products simply because they do not know enough about vegetable proteins.

Of course, habit plays a major role here because most of us have grown up eating animal products, and we feel something is lacking in our diet without them. I am not going to argue against the use of animal products. I am not a vegetarian myself, and I do not feel it is necessary for anyone to go to these lengths to be healthy. However, it does seem wise to limit the amount of animal protein in the diet to (perhaps) two ounces a day, in order to prevent an excessive build-up of nitrogen-containing compounds in the body. Again, people with type O blood might be the exception.

Now, we come to the question of balancing of protein. Protein is composed of amino acids, and there are certain amino acids that the human body does not manufacture, so they must be obtained from foods. If all of the amino acids are not present in the diet, the human body cannot build adequate protein.

It is believed that there are eight essential amino acids the body cannot manufacture, and many others that are used for specific protein synthesis, and which can be manufactured by the body from the eight essential ones. All eight essential fatty acids are found only in a few types of proteins, primarily in animal proteins, but they are also found in soy products. Thus, combining certain natural sources of protein creates a complete protein. Such combinations include beans with rice, corn, or some other grain, and some combinations of nuts and seeds with grains. There have been whole books written on the subject of protein combining. However, it is now realized by nutritionists that it is not absolutely essential that all eight essential amino acids be present in one meal, so if you obtain your protein from a variety of vegetable sources, likely all of the essential amino acids will find their way into your body through one source or another.

Soybeans have been widely touted as a savior of mankind in the area of protein nutrition, because soybeans are quite high in protein and contain all eight essential amino acids. Unfortunately, eating soybeans alone without other foods can be difficult to digest. They actually contain a substance that inhibits protein-digesting enzymes in the body. Asian cultures have been wise enough to experiment with soybeans over the centuries, and they have developed certain fermented foods that are much more readily digested, including tofu, tempeh, miso, and tamari. These are highly nourishing foods, and I recommend them to people who wish to ensure adequate protein in their diet without subjecting themselves to the extremes of concentrated protein and saturated fats present in most animal products.

The most important factor in eating protein is being able to digest and assimilate it. Otherwise, you will not be able to utilize it for repair and growth. If you have problems with "heartburn," intestinal gas, or other distress after eating protein foods, then you are probably suffering from a deficiency of digestive enzymes and/or hydrochloric acid in the stomach, and you may need temporary supplementation to get your system working better. If you have gas in your intestines after eating beans, try using Beano. This product contains a natural digestive enzyme that can help prevent gas from beans before it starts. See your nutritional health consultant or other professional for further guidance.

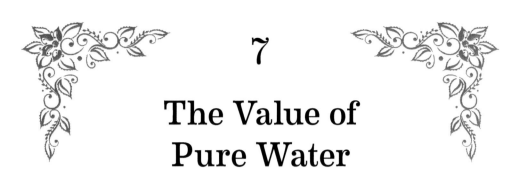

7

The Value of Pure Water

Pure water is an extremely important part of your diet. You cannot cleanse toxins out of your body without adequate amounts of pure water. Drink at least four glasses of pure water each day. Your need for water will vary but never let yourself get dehydrated. If you are tired, you may need more water.

Let's take a look at the simplest concept of good drinking water. Drinking water should ideally be free of all toxins, because one of its functions is to cleanse the body of waste matter. However, ideally, drinking water can also provide necessary nutrients.

Some studies have been done of particular societies wherein some members of the population live to an unusually advanced age. These are cultures in which the average life span is short because they live under difficult circumstances. However, those who survive to adulthood often live to be quite productive into advanced old age. These cultures include the Hunzas on the northern Indian peninsula, and the peoples of the Caucasus Mountains at the border between Europe and Asia. Many studies have been done regarding the food these people eat, in an attempt to determine what type of diet might be responsible for their prolonged vitality. However, if you compare various groups of people who have great vitality among their older members, you will find there is little in common in their diet. What they do have in common is that their drinking water comes from glacial streams.

Glacial water is pure distilled rainwater that has come down as snow and formed an ice pack. So we start with basically distilled water. However, the water is then tumbled down mountain streams through rocks in a highly turbulent manner, during which the water picks up a colloidal suspension of minerals. So, what these people are actually drinking is richly mineralized water in which the minerals are in colloidal form. *Colloidal* refers to minute particles that are kept in suspension, although they are not soluble by negative or positive electric charges on the particles.

Minerals are actually absorbed in the body better in a colloidal form than they are as soluble salts. It has been known for years that actual soluble minerals cannot be taken in easily by the body, but must be combined with organic materials or in colloidal form to be utilized effectively. So these people are evidently getting a rich source of mineral supplementation in their drinking water.

This type of water is not available easily to a person living in an urbanized area of the country. Various attempts have been made to synthesize this type of drinking water. In theory, one could do this by taking pure distilled water stored in glass, and adding to it a colloidal suspension of minerals. Never drink distilled water in plastic bottles because it picks up chemicals from the plastic. Distilled water, in general, is not a good source of drinking water because it is so deficient in minerals that it can dissolve and remove minerals from your body.

Avoid carbonated waters as they contain carbon dioxide, which produces carbonic acid in the body and dissolves out even more minerals.

Unfortunately, there is no good source of drinking water available to most of the clients that I have counseled on nutrition. Water is, of course, the basis of all life. It is one of the major ingredients of living systems, and the fact that there is no good source of pure water easily available is a shocking indictment of our present social structure.

Almost all public water sources are chlorinated. Indeed, they have to be, legally, in order to get any kind of financial support for the water systems constructed by cities. The amount of chlorine that is left in the water after it has been through a water treatment plant is inadequate to kill any new disease organisms that are introduced into it; otherwise, so much chlorine would be necessary that the water coming out of the tap would taste like Clorox! Actually, in some cities tap water does taste like bleach.

The chlorine that reacts with the organic compounds present in the water after treatment produces *chlorinated hydrocarbons*. They are highly toxic, and many of them are carcinogenic (cancer-causing). These compounds are present in public drinking water. These are thought to be a significant source of cancer-causing elements in the water supplies of some major cities, including cities located at the lower end of the Mississippi River that obtain their water from the river. This water has been recycled many times through various water systems, and it contains many waste products that react with chlorine to produce dangerous chemical compounds. Obviously, water that has been chlorinated or contains chlorine residue is not safe to drink.

One of the ways to get rid of chlorinated hydrocarbons is to filter the water through an activated carbon filter before drinking it. This removes any organic materials, which are absorbed into the activated charcoal. Many households have a filter on the tap from which drinking water is drawn. The filter simply passes the water through activated carbon. This is certainly better than no water treatment at all. However, it does carry with it certain dangers. Bacteria often attach to the carbon of the filter and start to grow on the organic compounds that are being filtered out of the water. People who drink water from which the chlorinated hydrocarbons have been removed, but to which bacteria and bacterial toxins have been added, are likely to have problems with their digestive tract.

A further complication of home water filters is that silver has been added to the carbon filter. This type of filter is known as a *silver-impregnated* carbon filter. The silver acts as a bacteria static ingredient, that is, it prevents the bacteria in the water from growing on the organic materials that are caught in the filter. However, there are other problems with this method. Primarily the fact that silver can interact with the chlorine compounds being filtered out of the water, producing silver chloride, which we then drink. This might or might not be harmful to the human digestive tract, depending upon your point of view, but it certainly is an added element the body was not designed to cope with.

There are many other types of filtration systems. Reverse osmosis removes virtually all of the organic compounds and salts from the water. Water softening elements remove calcium and other hard minerals, but replace them with salt, which is undoubtedly detrimental to the body. There are many, many varieties of filtration systems now available. They all have their claims and counterclaims, and it is difficult to evaluate them.

Certainly one of the most controversial of the claims that is being made by companies that set up entire household filtration systems is that the major amount of the water taken in by the human body is absorbed through the skin, and therefore filtering only your drinking water has little effect. This is somewhat controversial, and there is evidence on both sides.

Until such time as truly pure water is available, I recommend you drink spring water that is fairly rich in soluble minerals, if available. The next best available drinking water would be reverse osmosis-treated water, but certainly you would need to take a good mineral supplement while using this type of water, because reverse osmosis treatment leaches out all of the minerals.

8

Your Immune System

You are living in the middle of World War III and you are almost defenseless. Digging trenches or building bomb shelters isn't going to do you a bit of good, because you are fighting against weapons you can't even see. You haven't got much of a chance to fight back because you don't know who or what the enemy is—although there are speculations ranging from the Russians to General Mills to the American Medical Association.

Your life and health, and that of your children and their children to come, are at stake. In fact, what's actually at stake is the future of civilization on this planet—and that means *your* future. So it would be best to begin taking steps to protect yourself and win the "war" on a personal level.

The threat of AIDS and other infectious diseases has created a climate of fear throughout the world. It has also educated a lot of people as to what their immune system is and what it does. If you talked about the immune system thirty years ago, most people would give you a blank stare. Now, everyone knows about T-cells and white blood cell counts and antibody levels. Unfortunately, that doesn't mean they know how to protect themselves by building a strong immune system.

The war against the immune system might or might not have been started deliberately. Although there are many that view history from a conspiratorial point of view, it really doesn't matter to me whether we consider this started as a conspiracy or it was an accident brought on by stupid people who believed chemical innovations would improve the planet upon which we have lived for so long without the "benefit" of modern chemical processes. While the source of the war on the human immune system might be important in finding out how to "pick off your enemies," it's not that important in safeguarding your immediate health and that of your family.

As a child, I was brought up in the dawn of the new chemical era by parents who believed in having the most modern lifestyle for the benefit of their children. So we were raised on margarine, which was new and therefore undoubtedly better than butter, canned infant formula, frozen vegetables, bleached white flour, and other wonderful conveniences of modern life.

I was also always sickly as a child (guess why!), and my father, being a medical doctor, treated me with the latest miracle drugs to help get me over the infections and other illnesses that constantly plagued me. I remember sucking on penicillin lozenges like candy. They were supposed to help my chronic sore throats. They never did anything for the sore throats, but they might have contributed to my tonsils being taken out at an early age.

By the time I reached college, a good part of my hair was grey, I had a heart murmur, and I was routinely in the school infirmary every two weeks for several days with the latest bug that was going around. I had absolutely no resistance to any kind of infection.

You might say that I was one of the early victims of the war against the immune system. However, I fought back. There were a number of people among my college buddies who were quite interested in the possibility of obtaining better health through nutrition—an idea that was quite radical at the time and considered ludicrous by most scholars.

Adelle Davis was the only person talking about nutrition and health back then. She was widely regarded by many as being on the fringe and unscientific, although later her books became incredibly popular and many revered her approach. I learned to cook from her cookbook and discovered there was such a thing as whole-wheat flour—I hadn't known about it before. So, I began to bootstrap my way up to better health.

One of the basic things we need to understand in learning to protect the immune system is that all life forms on this planet are related. Obviously, this does not mean you are the same as a bacterium, but it does mean you have certain life processes that are quite similar, including the ways you produce energy.

The other principal idea for consideration is that most of the modern chemical innovations that have been hailed as forms of progress in our society are actually new ways of killing. For example, let us take a look at antibiotics. Antibiotics have been hailed as the savior of mankind. They have wiped out diseases that threatened to destroy whole groups of humans. Antibiotics are simply a way to kill bacteria without killing the human being infected by the bacteria. It is fairly common knowledge now that antibiotics can save us from various bacterial diseases, but they have also created major health problems by producing stronger strains of certain bacteria. They also destroy beneficial bacteria in the human intestines, thereby allowing harmful organisms to grow and create other health problems.

Another example is insecticides. Originally considered the salvation of agriculture, insecticides have proved to be a major scourge of our time. They create environmental havoc. Insecticides, of course, are designed to kill insects that reduce the amount of food that can be harvested. Insects also spread disease and reduce the profit of an agricultural enterprise. Insecticides, as poisons, were designed specifically to get around the immune system of the insect. It's something the insect doesn't "know" will harm it, and therefore the body does not put up defenses against the particular chemical.

From the first principle stated above—that all life forms on this planet have certain metabolic similarities—we can see that insecticides, in all likelihood, are poisons for humans, and indeed this is true. Although there are standards for how much pesticide you can use without causing obvious symptoms to the human population, this totally ignores the fact that these insidious chemicals are getting into our bodies, and by the nature of their design they remain in the system for many, many years—possibly a lifetime—as systemic poisons.

Antibiotics and pesticides are just two examples of the literally millions of chemicals with which we are poisoning our immune systems every day. What are the results?—cancer, allergies, auto-immune diseases, arthritis, millions of lost work hours because of colds and flu, and AIDS, which is just one of many scourges that threaten to destroy civilization. I am not saying that antibiotics and pesticides cause AIDS. But it is quite clear that someone with a weakened immune system is going to be much more susceptible to any kind of bacterial or viral infection that comes around.

All of the ailments listed above are defects in the effectiveness of the immune system. They are the results of it being too weak to respond properly to a challenge from the environment, such as an infectious disease organism. This is frightening, because the function of the immune system is to protect us from invading disease organisms. If we had no immune system, every time we cut ourselves our body would start to literally rot in that area. A single injury could kill us. If our immune systems are destroyed, there will be no human life on this planet. So what kind of insanity is it for industries—and even government agencies that are supposed to protect the public—to unleash millions of chemicals that end up destroying the human immune system? How did this occur? What are we going to do about it?

How can you win this war for yourself and your family? The only way is for each individual to take a stand and say "No" to the destruction around us, and to do everything possible to provide our bodies with valuable nutrition that can help protect the immune system.

The Immune System and
Indoor Environmental Hazards

Many people are aware of the hazards posed by smog, excessive exposure to sunlight, and other forms of pollution. However, there is often a greater possibility of immune system damage from the indoor environment than outdoors.

Many people work and/or live in "modern" buildings with no windows, central air-conditioning (which can become infected with mold), banks of fluorescent lights, and, quite often, new furnishings, including carpets loaded with formaldehyde.

Most of us live in a sea of pollutants that are eating away at the functioning of our immune systems. Fluorescent lights have been known for many years to destroy an excessive amount of Vitamin A in an individual exposed to them for long periods of time. They also put out ten-hertz radiation, which is damaging to the immune system. In addition, there is no doubt that the absence of natural spectrum light in fluorescent lighting can cause damage to the pituitary gland and a lowered functioning of much of the endocrine system.

A lack of fresh air is another hazard of the indoor environment. Fresh air is not just a romanticized term. Truly fresh air is high in negative ions, which are also found near waterfalls, the ocean, and in places where there is a high concentration of trees and other plants. These natural elements all produce negative ions, and it has been shown that a high concentration of negative ions in relationship to the number of positive ions in the air can be beneficial to the function of the immune system.

People who live in an atmosphere containing a high concentration of positive ions are often susceptible to chronic digestive disorders, headaches, and low immune system function, as well as frequent emotional depression. Just as the ratio of negative ions to positive ions is *increased* by the presence of living plants and moving water, it is dramatically *decreased* by central air-conditioning, which tends to put a lot of positive ions into the air. Therefore, people who work in an environment where there is central air-conditioning and who do not have a window they can open often suffer health problems.

In addition to problems with air-conditioning and no windows, an office environment that is designed to be attractive and comfortable often contains new furnishings. This is the worst thing that can be done for the immune systems of the employees who work in the office. New fabrics, such as those found in carpeting and draperies, release formaldehyde and other chemicals into the air for years after they've been installed—unless, of course, all-natural building materials are used, such as wool carpets. These poisons are detrimental to the body's detoxifying mechanisms, and they can lead to liver and immune system damage. New paint and wallpaper also outgas chemicals to which many people are sensitive, and which can cause subtle damage to the immune system, even in those people who do not have an obvious reaction.

Many employers who wish to attain maximum productivity from their employees are now replacing standard fluorescent light bulbs with full-spectrum bulbs such as Vita-Lite Full-Spectrum Lights or Kiva Lighting. These are relatively expensive lighting fixtures; however, employee productivity has risen dramatically when they are installed. Many business managers feel they are rewarded for the cost of the lights by increased employee productivity and the decrease in sick leave days.

Negative ion generators can be installed in offices to reduce the effect of central air-conditioning on the positive-negative ion balance. A wise business owner would probably choose a building with windows that can be opened by employees, if they care to do so, and where "old fashioned" room air-conditioners are used, rather than central air-conditioning. These small units produce fewer positive ions than central air-conditioning, because the positive ions are largely produced by the travel of air through long metal conduits.

The issues with chemicals off-gassing from new furnishings, fabric, and paint can often be ameliorated by the precautions recommended above, particularly being able to open the windows and allow rooms to air out when the weather permits. Offensive synthetic fabrics might well be avoided, if possible. Certainly, if you are going to have your office or home painted, it would be best to do it well before you plan to occupy the space, in order to give the paint fumes time to fully evaporate.

9

What Can I Eat?

This is a fairly common question that many people ask when they first embark on a nutritional program. They feel there are so many forbidden foods in their conventional diet that they are left with a choice between changing their lifestyle completely and starving. The intention here is not to create a situation in which starving is an essential part of your nutritional program! We certainly want you to provide your body with the food it needs to get well and stay well, without allowing yourself to get extremely hungry.

Unfortunately, this is not easy in our present culture. We live in a society that has become so highly commercialized that food is no longer considered a source of nutrition, but a subject for advertising and profit to the food industries. This is an unusual situation in historical terms, because even up to fifty years ago there was no such thing as a "food industry." There were certainly food traders and wholesalers, but the concept of taking foods and creating a processed product that could be commercialized and exploited for its profit-making potential had not entered into the American capitalistic scene.

So, now we have a culture in which food does not have as its primary purpose the nourishment of the body. For someone who is looking to regain good health, or to maintain good health, it is quite difficult to obtain food that contributes to this goal in a society in which food is considered primarily a way to make money, lots of it!

One of the first questions I ask of someone who is embarking on a nutritional program is: Do you cook for yourself? If the answer is

"Yes," then it is feasible to take this individual and educate him in the methods of preparing his own food so it is nourishing and contributes to his nutritional program. However, if he feels it is totally impossible for him to either take the time or learn to produce nourishing food in the kitchen, then it becomes much more difficult to set up a nutritional program for this individual.

The "natural food movement" has provided many options, and there are many restaurants and specialty stores that cater to people who are seeking good health through nutrition. However, for those of you who have not had the fortune and opportunity to find natural food restaurants nearby, you must learn to cook for yourself. The recipes in Part II will help you greatly in this regard.

So, let's begin with some basic principles about how to obtain nourishing food.

First, let's talk about food selection. Freshness is critical in choosing food that will promote health. As long as you are using food that has been preserved, packaged, canned, frozen, boxed, or even let sit on the shelf for a long period of time, you are not going to bring home food that will contribute the maximum to your health.

Let me enter here a word of caution because, unfortunately, many people who get involved in attempting to live on a healthy diet learn about food preservatives first, and they enthusiastically buy food items with labels that say "No Preservatives." This has become a catchword for the health food industry, and you will often see it in big letters on a package as an advertisement that this is something quite good for you. Preservatives were originally developed and put into food because food gets stale sitting on the grocery store shelf for long periods of time. Therefore, if you buy such a food, you need to make sure the food is fresh. Just because it says "No Preservatives" does not mean that it's fresh. I have seen many items sitting on the shelves of health food shores with labels such as this, when, in reality, the food items were stale or rancid when the package was opened.

As an ultimate food consumer, you have a responsibility to learn how to judge when a food is fresh or not. This is not just a matter of "does it taste good," because, unfortunately, many of us have gotten so used to eating stale food that we have become unaware of the changes in the taste of food as it gets older.

One of the most dangerous things you can do to your body—and I will go so far as to say it contributes to early aging, cancer and other major health problems—is to eat oils that have become rancid. This happens quite easily; for example, if you buy a bag of corn chips that have been fried in oil, placed in a plastic bag, and left out in the light, most of the time the oil in them will have become rancid. Please see Chapter 5 "Diet for Optimum Health" for more information about oils.

Other foods are much easier to judge. If vegetables are not fresh, they wilt. Unfortunately, in most grocery stores, vegetables that are left on the shelf overnight are freshened with sprays of water to which some preservatives have been added. So just because the vegetables look fresh does not mean you can buy them with impunity without knowing what the store is doing to them.

One of the nice things about buying fresh fruits and vegetables is that it is fairly easy to tell whether they are really fresh or not, and if you know how to select high quality fruits and vegetables, you can be assured of getting delicious and nourishing food every time you go to the grocery store or farmers' market.

Shopping for fresh fruits and vegetables is not automatically taught to people by their mothers at the grocery store anymore, so I often find they are unaware of how to choose fresh produce. If you really look at what you are buying and observe whether it looks fresh, or if it looks like it has been banged around too much in transit, or the leaves are wilted, or it looks like it came from a sick plant to begin with, then you have a good chance of getting high quality produce.

In selecting fresh fruits and vegetables, there is really no substitute for experience and using your own sense of taste. As your diet becomes more natural and with fewer artificially strong flavors, such as salt and sugar, your sense of taste will become more aware of the subtle aromas of fresh food, in comparison to food that has gone slightly stale. So, start with buying produce that looks the freshest and see how it tastes. If it doesn't taste good, go back to the store and try something else.

So, let's go back to the beginning. The most important thing about the food you eat is that it is fresh and intact. If you eat fresh, whole grains, and vegetables as the main staples of your diet—and supplement them with small quantities of concentrated proteins such as fish, tofu, poultry, beans, eggs, and red meats—then you will have a diet that stabilizes your body and spirit as you strive to achieve healing and perfect health. A lifelong nutritious diet will also support you in your quest for immortality!

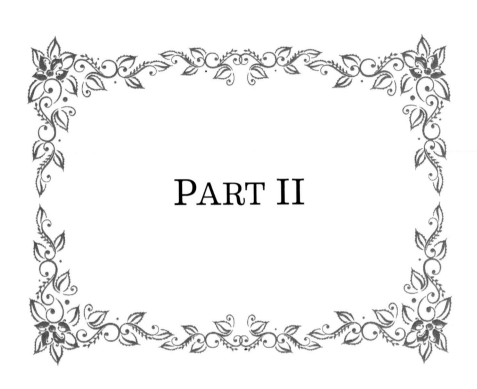

PART II

10

The Recipes

The First Ingredients

There are two key ingredients to preparing health-giving foods that you and your family will find delicious. The first of these is love. If you don't love the people you are preparing food for, including yourself, how are you going to take the time and attention required to select the highest quality ingredients and prepare them, while preserving all possible nutrients?

Food preparation requires a certain amount of knowledge and attention. It does not require magic. Those people who are supposedly "born cooks" are actually people who are interested enough to learn how to cook food well. They also have a good sense of taste and smell. Fortunately, these senses will be rehabilitated as you get excess sugar and salt, adulterated fats, and toxic chemicals out of your diet.

The second key ingredient is adventure. Taste and smell your food as you are preparing it; try different seasonings and approach cooking as a great adventure. You will open up a new world of artistry for your creative expression. Yes, you will have some failures, but you will learn. The reward will be turning your food into something that *you* have control over and that will contribute to your health as well as your eating pleasure.

The way to reduce the number of failures in this adventure is to look for the highest quality ingredients. If you want to experience what really fresh food tastes like, try buying your fresh vegetables and fruit from a farmer's market. Also purchase whole grains and flours at least once so you can taste the difference for yourself. You might even decide to purchase your own small flourmill to use at home. Once you have tasted truly fresh food with no added ingredients, you won't want to buy anything else.

How to Use These Recipes

When you start your nutritional program, you can prepare yourself for faster progress, less fatigue, and other reactions by taking the stress off your liver and digestive tract. The easiest way to do this is to go on a modified, protein sparing fast for a brief period. Protein shakes are a pleasant way to do this part of the program.

The first section includes protein shakes, green drinks, and other "cleansing foods." These foods will help to take a load off your liver and get your body ready to start eliminating toxins and pathogens. This part of the program should not last more than two weeks, but you might want to use these recipes forever. Green drinks and shakes are quick, energizing snacks and occasional meal substitutes that can be packed with good nutrients and still help remove toxins from your body.

The section on sweets is lengthy. We know that people on a strict nutritional program often feel deprived because they cannot eat sweets. We have found that maple syrup is the best sweetener for most people because it actually kills Candida, an extremely common fungal infection; whereas, all other sweeteners feed the fungus. This does not mean that you should automatically eat these desserts. If you tend to have high blood sugar, or have been diagnosed with actual diabetes, you must get your pancreas in good condition before you eat sweets.

It is critical that you avoid refined sugar, molasses, honey, fructose, fruit juice sweeteners, artificial sweeteners, and all other concentrated sweets when you start the program. If you have no sign of a fungal infection, you may be able to eat barley malt syrup or brown rice syrup, and we have included one recipe, for pecan pie, that we think tastes better with barley malt syrup than with maple syrup.

AN IMPORTANT NOTE ABOUT EATING MEAT: There is nothing wrong with eating red meat, chicken, and fish in moderation. However, when first beginning a detoxification diet it would be best to avoid meat for the first few weeks, and then add it back into your regular diet. The recipes that follow do not include meat because they are intended as the basis for detoxification, however, you can add meat or fish at your discretion. This would be primarily in the soup and grain recipes.

Enjoy these recipes in good health. Start by making your kitchen comfortable, because eating well and being healthy mean spending a lot of time in the kitchen. Restaurant food will never be as good as the food you create in your own kitchen, and it will never empower you in the same way cooking delicious, healthy food for yourself and your family will. If you don't enjoy spending time in the kitchen, take a look at the reasons why and find a remedy. Put a comfortable chair in a corner of your kitchen for guests and family to sit and chat while you cook, or you can use it yourself to rest while you wait for water to boil or to consult a recipe book. Put a portable radio on top of your refrigerator and listen to the news or play your favorite music. It's amazing how quickly dinner will be prepared while singing along to Patsy Cline's Greatest Hits. Do whatever must be done to make the kitchen comfortable. Make it the center of your household. Make sure you have a window to look out of, and brighten the room by growing herbs or other plants in it.

Besides comfort, an efficient kitchen will make your life easier. Have kitchen items that really work for you. A blender that can easily prepare smoothies every day is a necessity. A food processor will significantly reduce food preparation time. If you plan on baking, an electric mixer is invaluable. Make sure your knives are really sharp. A good sharp chopping knife is essential. You will use it every day. Little things, such as can openers that are easy to use, can make a real difference. Include a good selection of stainless steel cookware, a large soup pot, a small saucepan, big and small sauté pans, and a wok if you stir-fry a lot. Your needs may vary from other people, as do your tastes and diet, but make sure everything you use works. What's the point of having a dishwasher that doesn't clean the dishes or a can opener that takes ten minutes and lots of frustration to work properly. Don't be stingy with your kitchen utensils. The money you save by cooking at home and the benefits to your health will more than compensate for any extra expense.

Healthy eating comes from having a healthy relationship with the food you eat. Smell the produce you buy. Every day you should cook at least one meal for yourself, ideally all meals. Eating and cooking involve all the five senses: taste, smell, touch, sight, and sound, as well as a spiritual sense. Indulge these senses by buying the most delicious, aromatic, ripe, and beautiful fruits and vegetables you can find. High quality produce might cost more, but it will always be healthier than eating out.

The more you cook at home, the easier it will be, and you will become more and more organized, efficient, and creative. Explore the passion for food that comes naturally with a passion for life!

11

Basic Foods

❧ ALMOND MILK ❧

This is quite a tasty drink that's good with cereal, in blender drinks, or as a hot drink at bedtime. It is high in calcium and protein.

1 cup apple juice
1 cup water
½ cup raw almonds
2 tablespoons barley malt syrup or maple syrup
A few drops of sesame or almond oil

1. Put these ingredients in a blender. Blend on high speed for 2 minutes. Then pour through a strainer and scrape the remaining solids back into the blender.

2. Add 2 cups water

3. Blend on high speed for 1 minute. Pour through the strainer and mix with the other liquid. Simmer in a pan for 10 minutes, cool, and refrigerate.

4. What is left in the strainer at this point is mostly almond bran. Do not cook it, as it contains valuable enzymes that digest parasites in the intestines. Mix it with your children's cereal to help keep them from getting parasites, or eat it yourself.

The pineapple juice in this drink contains acids that break down the cell walls of the greens. Therefore the nutrients of the greens go directly into your body. Use green drink immediately after making. Play around with this recipe until you find a combination of ingredients that works for you. Be sure to taste the drink while making it. Let your taste buds tell you when it's ready to serve. The mint is quite nice but not necessary.

3 tablespoons frozen pineapple juice concentrate, or
$\frac{1}{2}$ cup fresh or frozen pineapple chunks
4 cups packed greens such as romaine, leaf lettuce,
and butter lettuce
$\frac{1}{4}$ to $\frac{1}{2}$ cup greens such as, spinach, watercress,
beet greens, dandelion, and arugula
1 to 2 sprigs mint

Place all ingredients in a blender and process until smooth.

Shakes

Here are some shake recipes to start out with. Get creative. You can put in anything you like. Try any other fresh or frozen soft fruits such as, papaya, pears, or pineapple. After 1 week the green mix can be increased as desired. The sprout powders, green powders, and protein powders (UltraClear is my favorite) are products that are quite beneficial.

❧ FLAX OIL SHAKE ❧

½ tablespoon flax seed oil
½ tablespoon sprout powder
½ tablespoon green powder
½ cup water
½ cup apple juice
½ banana
5 oz. (about 1 cup) frozen organic strawberries

Blend all ingredients until smooth.

❧ PROTEIN POWDER SHAKE ❧

2 heaping tablespoons protein powder
½ tablespoon sprout powder
½ tablespoon green powder
½ cup water
½ cup apple juice
½ banana
5 oz. frozen strawberries
½ cup frozen mango chunks

Blend all ingredients until smooth.

❧ ENERGY SHAKE ❧

½ tablespoon flax seed oil
2 heaping tablespoon protein powder
½ tablespoon sprout powder
½ tablespoon green powder
½ cup water
½ cup apple juice
½ cup frozen mango chunks
½ cup blueberries

Blend all ingredients until smooth.

12

Soups

❧ LENTIL SOUP ❧

(Serves 6 or can be lunch for a whole week)

3 small potatoes
3 medium carrots
3 stalks celery
1 medium onion
2 medium parsnips (optional)
5 cloves garlic
$\frac{1}{3}$ cup sesame oil
$\frac{1}{2}$ teaspoon each marjoram, savory, parsley, thyme
$\frac{1}{8}$ teaspoon celery seed
1 cup brown lentils
1 bay leaf
4 cup water or broth
3 teaspoons tamari
$\frac{1}{2}$ teaspoon sea salt
2 cup cooked brown rice

1. Wash and coarsely chop all vegetables, onions and garlic. In large soup pot, heat oil on medium. When hot, add onions and garlic and sauté for a few minutes. Add herbs and salt and sauté a few minutes longer.

2. Place lentils in a strainer and rinse well. Add lentils to vegetables along with the water or broth. Stir, cover and bring to a

boil. Reduce heat to medium, and allow to simmer for 30 minutes. When lentils are tender, add tamari and rice or serve over rice. Add more tamari to taste.

❧ MISO SOUP ❧

This nourishing soup can be made quite quickly with just a few ingredients. Miso soup is a delicious, satisfying addition to sandwiches, or eat it for breakfast on chilly mornings. For a heartier dish add a cup of cooked brown rice or barley. The flavor of miso is great without the shiitake mushrooms, but they are a delicious addition if you have them.

> 2 cups, plus 4 cups pure or filtered water
> 3 to 4 dried shiitake mushrooms, (optional)
> 1 to 2 blocks tofu, cubed small
> 1 small bunch broccoli, green beans, kale, or other greens
>   cut into bite-size pieces
> 2 ½ tablespoons mugi (barley) miso

Garnish:
2 green onions, chopped small
Toasted sesame oil

1. Bring 2 cups water to a boil. Place dried shiitake mushrooms into a bowl. Pour boiling water over, and allow to soak for 15 minutes.

2. Place remaining 4 cups water along with tofu into a medium soup pot, cover and bring to a boil. Reduce heat and stir to separate any tofu that has stuck together. Cover and allow to simmer gently for 10 minutes.

3. Remove mushrooms from water and slice into strips, discarding stems. Add mushrooms along with mushroom broth to tofu mixture.

4. Using a teacup remove about ½ cup of water from pot. Add miso to teacup and mix with a fork until there are no lumps. Return miso mixture to pot stirring in well. Add green vegetable and allow to simmer for 3 minutes (do not boil), or just until the green vegetable is at the height of its color.

5. Remove from heat. Garnish each bowl with green onions and a dash of toasted sesame oil.

✑ BORSCH ✎

Borscht is a delicious and super-nutritious way to eat winter root vegetables. There are endless variations for preparing borscht but this one encourages you to use the entire beet, greens, stems and all. Optional ingredients add flavor and nutrients but aren't necessary for a great tasting soup.

1 yellow onion
2 cloves garlic
2 tablespoons butter
2 tablespoons any whole grain flour
I teaspoon dill
1 bay leaf
1 teaspoon sea salt
7 cup pure or filtered water, vegetable cooking water, or broth
4 to 5 large or 6 to 7 smaller beets, plus greens and stems
1 large carrot
1 large potato
1 small turnip, (optional)
1 small parsnip, (optional)
2 stalks celery
½ small head cabbage

2 tomatoes, or 1 tablespoon tomato paste
Juice of one half lemon (about 2 tablespoons)
Tamari to taste

1. Mince onion and garlic. In a large soup pot melt butter over medium heat. Add onion and sauté just until onion turns translucent. Add garlic and flour and cook stirring constantly for one minute. Slowly pour water or broth into flour mixture about a cup at a time stirring well after each addition. Add dill, bay leaf and salt, turn heat to high and bring to a boil.

2. Meanwhile, wash and trim vegetables. Remove greens and stems from beets and set aside for later. Thoroughly scrub dirt off all root vegetables. Using the grater attachment on your food processor, grate beets, potato, carrot along with turnip and parsnip, if using. If you prefer, finely chop vegetables into small pieces. Chop celery.

3. When broth has come to a boil, stir in grated vegetables and celery. Turn heat down to low and allow to simmer, covered, for about 10 minutes.

4. Chop cabbage thinly lengthwise removing the tough inner stem as you go. Then chop cabbage into thirds crosswise. Chop tomatoes into small pieces. Wash beet stems and leaves thoroughly removing any inedible or yellowed parts. Chop into small pieces and stir into soup pot along with cabbage and tomato or tomato paste. Cook 10 minutes longer.

5. Stir in lemon juice and add tamari to taste. Serve in large bowls with a dollop of sour cream or yogurt if you'd like. Have thick slice of whole grain bread handy on the side.

≈ CLASSIC JAPANESE HEALING SOUP ≈

This Japanese sea vegetable soup is super-nutritious and soothing.

7 cups pure or filtered water or vegetable cooking water
6 dried shiitake mushrooms
2 carrots, thinly sliced
2 stalks celery, thinly sliced
1 onion, diced
2 cloves garlic, diced
3 large leaves bitter greens such as kale or collards, chopped
1-inch piece daikon radish, diced
1 small bunch of fresh parsley, chopped
2 to 3 pieces dried wakame, soaked and chopped
    (discard soaking water)
Pinch of thyme
¼ pound tofu, cubed small
½ to 1 cup cooked brown rice
3 tablespoons mugi (barley) miso
1 teaspoon tamari

1. Soak shiitake mushrooms in 2 cups of pure or filtered water for
   20 minutes. Remove mushrooms and chop, discarding stems.
   In a large soup pot, combine mushrooms, mushroom soaking
   water, and 5 cups additional water. Bring to a boil and simmer
   10 minutes.

2. Add carrots, celery, onions and garlic Allow to simmer 10
   minutes more. Add chopped bitter greens, daikon, parsley,
   wakame, thyme, and tofu. Simmer 10 more minutes.

3. Using a teacup, remove about ½ cup of broth. Stir miso into
   broth until completely dissolved. Return to pot and add brown
   rice and tamari. Simmer 5 minutes being careful not to boil the
   miso. Eat immediately, seasoning with additional tamari,
   if desired.

∾ LEEK AND LENTIL SOUP ∾

This soup is savory and satisfying.

    1 tablespoon butter
    1 tablespoon olive oil
    1 large leek, white part only, chopped thinly
    1 onion, chopped small
    3 cloves garlic, minced
    1 teaspoon dried tarragon
    1 bay leaf
    ¼ teaspoon powdered fennel seed
    1 cup brown lentils, rinsed
    1 carrot, chopped
    2 potatoes, chopped (optional)
    6 cup vegetable broth

In a large soup pot, melt butter with olive oil over medium high heat. Lower heat slightly and add leeks and onion. Sauté, stirring frequently until softened, for about 5 minutes. Add garlic, tarragon, bay leaf, and fennel. Sauté for several minutes more. Add lentils, carrots, potatoes, and broth. Turn heat to high and bring soup to a boil. Reduce heat and simmer 25 minutes until lentils are tender.

∾ KITCHEN SINK VEGETABLE SOUP ∾

This soup, while needing a few basics, can be made with whatever vegetables are in season. Choose three or four items from the vegetables options list and as many other optional items as you'd like. By no means are these lists comprehensive. Be creative and patient. Take your time attractively chopping the vegetables, and give plenty of time to sautéing the onions. You can't rush a good soup. Soups freeze wonderfully and often taste ten times as good after thawing or after sitting two days in the refrigerator.

2 to 3 tablespoons cooking oil

1 chopped onion

½ teaspoon sea salt

3 to 4 minced cloves garlic

2 chopped carrots

2 chopped stalks celery

3 to 4 quartered new potatoes

10 cups of pure or filtered water or broth

2 bay leaves

2 teaspoons of any or all, basil, marjoram, thyme, sage, savory, oregano

Several tablespoons tamari, to taste

Optional Vegetables:

1 to 2 chopped tomatoes

2 to 3 sliced zucchini or other summer squash

1 head cauliflower pulled into flowerets

1 head of broccoli cut into flowerets with stem peeled and sliced

1 bag of frozen corn or peas

Several handfuls trimmed green beans

1 cup or more peeled, seeded and chopped winter squash

2 cups or more of chopped spinach or other leafy greens

Other Optional Ingredients:

1 to 2 cans cooked kidney or other beans

1 cup fresh chopped parsley leftover cooked rice or noodles leftover cooked lentils any other ingredient that strikes your fancy

1. Heat oil in a large soup pot on medium high. Add chopped onions and salt and sauté several minutes until onions have turned translucent and released their juices. Add garlic and herbs and sauté several minutes more. Add carrots, celery, and potatoes in stages sautéing a few minutes after each addition. Allow vegetables to cook several minutes before adding any liquid.

2. Add water or broth slowly a cup at a time stirring liquid and vegetable mixture gently together. When all liquid has been added, cover and allow to come to a low boil. Reduce heat and simmer for 20 minutes.

3. Prepare additional ingredients and add them in stages. Thicker, slower cooking vegetables such as broccoli stems or cauliflower should be put in several minutes before delicate ones such as spinach, which should be added at the last minute. Canned beans, rice or other cooked grains can be added at anytime in this last stage. Simmer until all pre-cooked ingredients are heated through. Add chopped parsley a minute or two before serving.

❧ WINTER SQUASH SOUP WITH COLLARDS ❧

This soup is sweet and rich and an excellent way to enjoy the delicious flavor of winter squash.

1 medium butternut, buttercup acorn squash, or other
    sweet winter squash
4 cup pure or filtered water or vegetable broth
3 tablespoons butter
1 to 2 teaspoons sea salt
1 medium yellow onion, chopped
2 cloves garlic, minced
2 teaspoons dried parsley
Small bunch collard greens
Tamari
Chopped fresh parsley for garnish (optional)

1. Using a large, sharp knife cut squash down the middle lengthwise. Scoop out seeds and reserve to wash and toast in the oven later.* Chop each squash half into quarters. Cut the fibrous

stem off the squash. Using a sharp paring knife or vegetable peeler remove the peel from each squash section. Chop squash into small chunks and set aside.

2. Melt butter in a large soup pot. Add the onion and sea salt and sauté until onion becomes translucent. Add the garlic and dried parsley and sauté one minute longer. Place squash along with water or broth into pot. Turn heat to high and allow to come to a boil, stirring occasionally. Reduce heat to low, cover, and allow to simmer 20 minutes until squash becomes tender and breaks apart easily.

3. Meanwhile, wash collards thoroughly discarding any yellowed leaves. Remove and discard the tough inner stem to each leaf. Chop leaves into small pieces.

4. When squash is tender, transfer half the soup into a blender and process until smooth. Return to pot and stir in. If you prefer, you can use a potato masher or slotted spoon to mash squash in the pot.

5. Stir collard greens into soup, and allow to simmer for 10 minutes longer until greens are bright and colorful.

6. Add tamari to taste. Just before serving, stir in a handful of fresh chopped parsley or use a few pinches of parsley to garnish each serving if you'd like.

*To toast squash seeds, wash them thoroughly removing any squash particles that cling to seeds. Spread seeds on a cookie sheet and sprinkle with sea salt. Toast in a 350°F oven until they become fragrant. Crack the seeds with your teeth and enjoy the delicious meat.

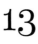

13

Whole Grains

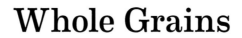

For most people, whole grains should be a major part of the diet. It is sad that our society has become dependent upon white flour products, which have little nutritive value and may contain toxins such as bleaches and dough conditioners, as well as pesticides and preservatives.

The world of whole grains is a rich one that can provide you with almost infinite variety in your diet. Brown rice tests as the best grain for a great many people, so we have included a number of recipes using it. But explore other whole grains, and you will be rewarded with pleasant experiences. Barley is a wonderful grain to add to soups and stews, and barley flour, because it contains little gluten, makes a good addition to pie crusts and cookies. Barley is an excellent grain for young children. I believe that it actually helps their immune systems to develop well. Very young children who can't eat grains are able to drink barley water (water drained from cooking barley) when added to their milk or juice drinks.

A word about pasta: It's a favorite American food, but white flour pasta has little nutritional value. People who try to substitute any whole-grain pasta off the health food store shelf in their recipes are often shocked by how little it resembles regular pasta. In the interest of saving you the "gooey or chewy" experience of some whole-grain pastas, I suggest you try the following list of excellent pastas. Definitely avoid pastas composed solely of brown rice flour, corn flour, or whole-wheat flour. Try these:

• De Bole's Whole-Wheat and Jerusalem Artichoke Spaghetti

- Ancient Harvest Quinoa and Whole-Wheat Spirals
- Spelt lasagna noodles
- Soba or buckwheat noodles
- Various sprouted kamut and spelt pastas

Breakfast Cereals

Cold breakfast cereals in a box are not the most nutritious way to eat grains. Far better are hot cereals that you prepare each morning. Some hot cereals that only take a few minutes to cook are:

- Barley Plus (Erewhon)
- Brown Rice Cream (Lundberg) and other similar brown rice cereals
- Mixed grain hot cereals available in health food stores

If you cook these cereals with extra water just until they are "soupy" you won't need to add milk. Just add a dab of butter and a little maple syrup. Another way to have a quick whole grain cereal is to reheat cooked grains such as brown rice or barley with milk, almond milk, butter, and/or maple syrup. Limit oatmeal or other oat cereals. Oats can contribute to Candida fungal overgrowth.

Grains

Below is the amount of water and time required to cook 1 cup of each grain. Add salt, as desired, to water before adding grain.

Barley:	3 cups, 1 hour 25 minutes
Brown Rice:	2 cups, 1 hour
Buckwheat:	2 cups, 15 minutes
Bulgur/	
Cracked Wheat:	2 cups, 15 to 20 minutes
Millet:	2 cups, 25 minutes

Wheat Berries:	3 cups, 2 hours
Wild Rice:	3 cups, 1 hour
Quinoa:	2 cups, 15 minutes

Flours

Barley: excellent mixed with equal parts whole-wheat pastry flour for pie crusts.

Brown Rice: good for crunchy cookies.

Buckwheat: mix equal parts with whole-wheat, spelt or kamut flour for pancakes.

Kamut: use like whole-wheat flour.

Millet: wonderful in pound cake.

Spelt: use like whole-wheat flour.

Whole-wheat: pastry flour and whole-wheat bread flour

❦ SIMPLE BROWN RICE ❦

There are almost as many ways to cook brown rice as there are varieties. This method yields a chewy rice that is not starchy. Be sure to purchase organic brown rice. Experiment with short grain, long grain, and fragrant basmati rice. Use this simple recipe to cook them all to perfection. For larger quantities, increase the amount of ingredients accordingly.

  1 cup rice
  1 ½ cups water
  ¼ teaspoon salt
  2 teaspoons oil or butter

1. Rinse rice well. Pour into a medium-size pot and add oil. Sauté on medium-high heat, stirring constantly, coating rice grains with oil and allowing the water to evaporate until rice is quite dry.

2. Meanwhile, in a separate saucepan, bring water and salt

to a boil.

3. When the rice is dry pour boiling water into pot over rice. Stir well to combine and cover. Reduce heat to low and allow it to simmer for 35 to 40 minutes. Check rice occasionally to make sure it doesn't burn, but do not stir.

4. When rice is chewy and has absorbed all the water remove from heat and keep covered until ready to use.

✌ DR. HUNTLEY'S FOOLPROOF RECIPE FOR DELICIOUS BROWN RICE ✌

This specific recipe makes delicious, perfect brown rice every time. It requires the use of a crockpot or rice steamer. Make sure yours is made of stainless steel on the inside, and not aluminum, which is a toxic metal.

> 2 teaspoons toasted sesame seed oil
> 1 ½ cup pure or filtered water
> ¼ teaspoon salt
> 1 ½ cup organic basmati and short-grain rice mixture

1. Fill a 4-quart sauce pan halfway with pure or filtered water. Put sesame oil in bottom of steamer and place on top of pot. Cover steamer and bring water to a boil.

2. Meanwhile, in a separate saucepan bring water and salt to a boil.

3. Clean rice by placing in a large bowl or measuring cup, covering with a generous amount of water and swishing. Pour into strainer to drain.

4. When both pots of water have come to a boil pour cleaned rice into steamer and pour boiling salted water on top of the rice. Lower heat to medium and steam 50 minutes or until done.

5. Stir rice and enjoy!

INGREDIENT TIP: Combine 2 parts organic short-grain brown rice to 1 part organic brown basmati and keep stored in an airtight container on a handy shelf for frequent usage.

✒ IVONNE'S BREAKFAST RICE ✒

(Serves 2)

A quick and delicious breakfast that is especially satisfying if you crave sweets; this cereal becomes a pudding in the refrigerator.

　1 cup cooked brown rice
　½ cup milk or almond milk
　Maple syrup, to taste
　1 teaspoon butter
　Dash cinnamon
　Dash nutmeg

Combine all ingredients in a small saucepan. Bring to a simmer and cook uncovered for ten minutes. Eat warm, topped with fresh fruit, if desired.

✒ BROWN RICE OR BARLEY DELIGHT ✒

　1 teaspoon sesame oil
　10 oz. package frozen organic corn
　2 chopped carrots
　2 to 3 cloves garlic, minced
　¼ teaspoon marjoram
　¼ teaspoon dill weed
　¼ teaspoon sea salt
　1 cup brown rice or barley
　1 ¾ cup pure or filtered water (add 1 extra cup if using barley)

1. Heat oil in a heavy saucepan on medium heat. Sauté the garlic, carrots, and corn for a minute or two. Add marjoram, dill weed, salt and rice (or barley) and sauté 3 minutes.

2. Meanwhile, in separate saucepan bring water to a boil. Pour boiling water into rice mixture, cover and allow to come to boil again. Reduce heat and allow to simmer for 30 minutes (50 minutes for barley), stirring occasionally.

3. At the end of cooking you may add for additional flavor: sea salt, tamari, or 1 teaspoon butter. Allow to sit covered for 1 minute. Serve.

❧ FRIED RICE ☙

(Serves 4)

This Thai-inspired fried rice makes a quick meal. If you prepare all the ingredients ahead of time it can be quite easy. A wok is the best choice if you have one. Skillet users will find the tricky part is to have the heat high enough to scramble the eggs quickly without burning the rice. If this is too difficult, scramble the eggs separately and mix in the rice and vegetables while the eggs are still a little soft. The measurements and ingredients in fried rice are deliberately vague. Add ingredients to your whims, tastes, and availability. Every pot of fried rice is different.

½ cake tofu
2 eggs beaten
Dash cayenne
Tamari
1 teaspoon toasted sesame oil
2 tablespoons sesame oil, plus 1 teaspoon
2 carrots thinly chopped on a diagonal
Handful frozen peas
Chopped greens
1 small zucchini cubed
Small head of broccoli peeled and separated into flowerets

2 cloves garlic, minced
2 cups leftover brown rice
2 green onions, chopped into one inch pieces
Handful cilantro, chopped
1 lime

1. Slice tofu into small ¼ inch cubes. Place in a small saucepan, cover with water and bring to a boil. Reduce heat slightly and continue to cook at a low boil covered for 10 minutes. Drain the tofu and rinse with cold water separating by hand any tofu cubes that have stuck together.

2. Meanwhile, beat the eggs with a couple dashes of cayenne and tamari to taste. Set aside.

3. Prepare all vegetables and have them readily accessible before beginning to stir-fry.

4. In a wok or large skillet heat 2 tablespoons sesame oil on medium heat. Add carrots and a pinch of salt. Stir-fry one minute until carrots brighten. Add zucchini and stir-fry 2 to 3 minutes more. Add garlic, peas, greens and broccoli and continue to stir-fry for a few minutes. Add tofu and stir-fry well into vegetables. Add the rice to the pan and mix in well. The pan or wok will become quite dry at this point. If you want to cook the eggs separately remove the rice and vegetable mixture from the pan. Heat 1 teaspoon of sesame oil for a few seconds then add the eggs and scramble. Just before the eggs have completely hardened add the rice and vegetable mixture back to the pan. Or:

5. Quickly make a large well in the middle of the rice scraping and piling the rice-vegetable mixture to the sides of the wok. Pour in 1 teaspoon sesame oil followed by the eggs. Scramble the eggs in the center until fairly well done avoiding as much of the rice and vegetables as possible. The drier the eggs the better

the fried rice. Quickly mix rice and eggs together generously seasoning with tamari, (about 3 to 4 tablespoons or more to taste,) and the toasted sesame oil. Add green onions stir one minute more and remove from heat.

6. Serve in large bowls with a few generous pinches of cilantro sprinkled on top and a large wedge of lime for squeezing.

⪻ TABOULI ⪼

1 cup bulgur (cracked whole-wheat)
1 ½ cup boiling water
Pinch salt
3 teaspoons tamari
⅓ cup olive oil
½ cup lemon juice
2 cloves garlic minced or pressed
3 cup chopped fresh parsley
2 to 3 chopped tomatoes (optional)
4 chopped green onions
½ large or small cucumber peeled and chopped small
¼ teaspoon allspice

1. Rinse bulgur and place in a large bowl. Pour boiling water over bulgur and let sit covered for about half an hour.

2. Add salt, tamari, olive oil and lemon juice to bulgur and let marinate several hours or overnight if you wish.

3. Add rest of ingredients and more tamari to taste. Serve.

PASTA WITH SPINACH AND TOASTED WALNUTS

½ cup walnuts
2 tablespoons olive oil
1 small onion, chopped
3 cloves garlic, chopped
¼ teaspoon sea salt
1 package of fresh spinach
Tamari to taste
8 oz. whole-wheat, sprouted grain, or other
     fettuccine or ribbons
Italian parsley for garnish

1. Place large pot of salted water on to boil for pasta.

2. Toast walnuts in a heavy skillet over medium heat stirring frequently to keep from burning. When darkened and fragrant remove from pan and set aside.

3. Add olive oil to skillet. Sauté onion with salt about 10 minutes, stirring frequently, until translucent. Add garlic. Stir and cook 2 to 3 minutes longer. Add spinach and sauté 8 minutes or so, stirring frequently until spinach is wilted; don't overcook.

4. Meanwhile cook pasta according to package directions for al dente, and drain. Rinse pasta under cold water to remove excess starch.

5. In a large bowl combine pasta, onion and spinach mixture, and walnuts. Add tamari to taste and toss. Garnish each serving with freshly chopped Italian parsley.

༈ SOBA NOODLES WITH KALE ༈

Soba noodles are a type of pasta from Japan made from buckwheat or brown rice available in most health food stores. This is a hearty fall or winter meal in one.

6 oz. soba noodles
2 tablespoons sesame oil
3 cloves garlic, minced
1 tablespoon fresh ginger, peeled and minced
¼ teaspoon dried red chili
3 large leaves kale, spines removed and coarsely chopped
1 green onion, thinly chopped on a diagonal
3 tablespoons tahini
1 tablespoon toasted sesame oil
1 tablespoon maple syrup
2 tablespoons tamari
2 teaspoons toasted sesame seeds*

1. Bring a large pot of water to boil. Add soba and cook according to package directions being careful not to overcook.

2. Meanwhile prepare kale, garlic and ginger. Toast sesame seeds and set aside. Drain soba and set aside.

3. In a small bowl combine tahini, toasted sesame oil, maple syrup, and tamari and set aside.

4. In a large skillet or wok, heat sesame oil on medium high. Add garlic, ginger, red chili, and kale and stir-fry constantly until kale begins to wilt and turn bright green. Stir in tahini mixture along with green onions. Add soba noodles and toss until noodles are warmed through. Sprinkle with sesame seeds and enjoy.

*Note: toast sesame seeds in a heavy skillet on medium heat until they become fragrant. (About 1 minute.)

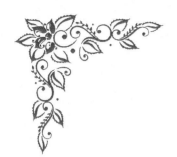
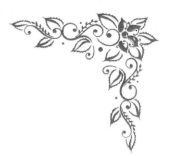

14

Proteins

During the first part of your nutritional program, you will be primarily removing toxins from your body. Excess protein in your diet inhibits this process, so I suggest you keep protein to a minimum in the beginning. Protein shakes, almond milk, tofu dishes, and, rarely, small amounts of animal products should be plenty of protein to supply your body's needs during detoxification.

As you get well along into the program and start rebuilding and repairing body structures, you will need much higher quantities of protein. At this stage, three to eight months into the program, you will probably start to crave animal protein. Eat it, but be sure to get meat that is from free-range animals that are fed natural foods without hormones, antibiotics, growth stimulants, and other feed additives. If you think beef from a regular grocery store is okay, read *Mad Cowboy* by Howard Lyman. Let me assure you that the way chickens are raised is even worse. When you learn what goes into the meats commonly sold in regular stores, you will not be surprised that cancer rates are skyrocketing.

Unfortunately, I cannot agree with those who advocate eating texturized soy protein "imitation meats." Soybeans, unless fermented, as in tofu or miso, can be quite difficult for most people to digest. The following recipes focus on tofu and other meatless proteins.

❧ TOFU WITH TAMARI AND LEMON ❧

(Serves 4)

High quality organic oils make this dish especially nutritious and delicious. It freezes well and can be easily reheated.

> 2 one-pound blocks firm tofu
> Barley flour for dredging
> Coconut oil
> Organic, refined sesame oil

Tamari-Lemon Sauce:
¼ cup toasted sesame oil
¼ cup tamari
¼ cup lemon juice
1 or 2 large cloves of garlic
¼ cup chopped fresh parsley (optional)
1 large chopped green onion (optional)
2 tablespoons toasted sesame seed (optional)

1. Preheat oven to 350°F.

2. Slice tofu in ¼ inch thick slices. Heat 1 tablespoon each coconut and sesame oils in a large heavy skillet on medium heat. While the oil is heating spread about ¼ cup flour on a plate to use for dredging. Make sure the oil is hot by dropping a pinch of flour in it and watching for it to sizzle. Dip tofu slices in the flour lightly coating each side and slide into hot oil cooking each side a couple of minutes until flour is browned. While the first four or five slices are browning dredge the second batch and continue in this manner until all the tofu has been browned. Add more flour to dredging plate or oil to pan as needed. Lay browned slices in a single layer in two large baking dishes; a cookie sheet or casserole can both work fine. Make sauce.

To Make the Tamari-Lemon Sauce:

1. Mince or press garlic and whisk all ingredients together. Adjust tamari to taste.

2. Pour sauce evenly over tofu and bake at 350°F for 15 minutes. Serve with brown rice. Or cool and freeze all, or a portion of the tofu, in an airtight container, separating tofu layers with wax paper.

❧ PESTO ❧

Makes enough pesto for 2 (16 oz.) packages of pasta.

This traditional-style pesto doesn't need the cheese to taste wonderful. Look for DeBoles Whole-wheat & Jerusalem Artichoke Pasta to serve this over. Be sure to use the freshest basil available with lots of small leaves and flowers. Use a high quality, fragrant olive oil.

1 cup walnuts, toasted or raw
2 large cloves garlic or more to taste, peeled and chopped
1 packed cup fresh basil leaves
⅔ cup olive oil
Sea salt to taste

1. Finely mince garlic. Chop walnuts into small pieces. Wash basil and remove leaves and flowers from the stems. Mince basil with a sharp knife or, even better, use your fingers to tear the leaves into tiny pieces. I've been told this is the real Italian way to prepare pesto. Purists believe a knife destroys some of the basil's aroma and flavor.

2. Combine walnuts, garlic and basil with the olive oil. Add a few pinches sea salt to taste. Toss with pasta. Delicious. You can also freeze pesto indefinitely for a quick dinner on some wintry eve.

❧ FRIED TOFU ❧

1 lb. block tofu allowed to drain 10 minutes in a strainer
½ tablespoon tamari
2 tablespoons lemon juice
1 tablespoon toasted sesame oil
¼ cup sesame oil

1. Combine tamari, lemon juice, and toasted sesame oil to make a marinade. Slice tofu crosswise and lengthwise into ½-inch cubes and place in a shallow dish or plate. Pour marinade over top tossing gently to coat. Allow to marinate at least 10 minutes or up to 2 days tightly covered and refrigerated.

2. In a large skillet, heat oil on medium. When oil is hot, add tofu, arranging in a flat layer so that tofu will brown evenly. Fry until bottom is lightly browned and crispy. Flip carefully turning each piece of tofu and brown other side. When other side is browned you can add to a stir-fry or cool and store in an airtight container in the refrigerator for up to 3 to 4 days.

❧ BASIC STIR-FRY WITH TOFU ❧

A wok is much easier for this recipe if you have one. Or you can use a large skillet but you may find yourself having to stir-fry the vegetables in two or more rounds.

The idea behind stir-frying is to keep the cooking time to a minimum so as to bring out the height of the vegetables' flavor, color and vitamin content. Generally, the brighter the color, the more nutritious is the vegetable. You should have all vegetables chopped beforehand and separated by what takes more time to cook and what takes less.

½ tablespoon coconut oil
1 large carrot
1 stem broccoli

¼ head cauliflower
½ cup shredded cabbage
A few slices of red pepper
½ cake fried tofu

For sauce, mix together:
1 tablespoon tamari
1 tablespoon lemon juice
1 tablespoon toasted sesame oil (Spectrum Naturals
    preferably)
1 clove garlic
¼ teaspoon minced fresh ginger

1. Scrub and slice carrot. Cut off broccoli top and separate into flowerets. Peel stem and slice thinly. Separate cauliflower into flowerets.

2. Prepare the vegetables by heating the oil over medium-high heat and begin to cook the vegetables when hot. Add vegetables in the following order, stir-frying for a minute before adding the next ingredient: cauliflower, carrots, cabbage, broccoli, tofu, and pepper. Pour on sauce and stir-fry until everything is bright and colorful but still crispy, a few minutes more after adding last ingredient. Serve over rice with tamari and toasted sesame seeds as condiments.

❧ SWEET AND SAVORY TOFU ❧

(Serves 4 to 6)

1 cake firm tofu
Sesame oil for frying
2 cups of 1 or more of these vegetables washed, trimmed,
    and attractively chopped:
Green beans
Broccoli
Carrots

Cauliflower
Celery
Chinese cabbage
Chinese broccoli
Green, red, or yellow pepper

Marinade:
¼ cup tamari
¼ cup pure or filtered water
2 tablespoons maple syrup
⅛ cup toasted sesame oil
3 to 4 dried shiitake mushrooms
1 to 1½ teaspoons mustard powder
1 tablespoon minced ginger
3 cloves minced garlic
Pinch crushed red chili (optional)
1 teaspoon arrowroot powder
Wine to taste (optional)

1. Drain tofu. Quarter tofu and cut each quarter into halves on a diagonal to form triangles. Lay each triangle long side down and cut into thirds forming three separate triangles. You will have 24 pieces.

2. In a small saucepan combine all sauce ingredients except arrowroot powder. Bring to a boil and simmer 15 minutes.

3. Lay tofu pieces in a single layer in a large container. Pour sauce over tofu and let marinate at least 1 hour or up to 2 days tightly covered in the refrigerator. The longer the tofu marinates the more flavorful it will become.

4. In a large skillet heat a scant ¼-inch of sesame oil on medium-low heat. When oil is hot, but not smoking, fry tofu in single layers until crispy on two sides.

5. Remove tofu from skillet with a slotted spatula and allow to drain on a plate lined with paper towels.

6. Pour off excess oil from pan and stir-fry prepared vegetables with ¼ cup of the marinade until vegetables are bright and crispy. Combine vegetables and tofu in a large bowl.

7. Remove shiitake mushrooms from marinade and slice into strips removing inedible stems. Add to vegetables and tofu.

8. Pour marinade into skillet reserving ½ cup in a cup. Bring marinade to a boil. Stir arrowroot powder into ½ cup of cold marinade making sure powder is completely dissolved. Whisk into boiling marinade continuing to whisk until sauce thickens. You may want to whisk in a little water if sauce is too thick or potent at this point, especially if you haven't used the wine.

9. Pour sauce over vegetables and tofu and serve over brown rice. Amazing!

⚘ CURRIED LENTILS WITH APPLE ⚘

Serve this slightly spicy dish with fragrant brown basmati rice and a cool salad to cut the heat from the spices.

1 cup lentils, rinsed
1 to 2 ½ cup pure or filtered water
1 small red onion, chopped
2 to 3 cloves garlic, minced
2 tablespoons sesame oil
Pinch each: allspice, coriander, cinnamon, cayenne, and cumin
¼ teaspoon thyme
⅛ teaspoon turmeric
1 teaspoon fresh ginger root
1 cooking apple, cored and chopped
Tamari to taste
Handful fresh cilantro, chopped, (optional)

1. Place lentils and pure or filtered water in a medium saucepan. Bring to a boil and then reduce heat to a simmer. Cover and allow to cook about 30 minutes, until lentils are tender.

2. Meanwhile, heat the oil in a skillet on medium-high. Add the onion and garlic and stir-fry for a few minutes. Stir in the spices and ginger root well into the onion and oil mixture and cook one minute longer.

3. Pour onion-spice mixture into the lentils and stir well to combine. Add tamari to taste, and allow to cook 10 minutes longer.

4. Add the apple a few minutes before removing from the heat. Add more tamari to taste and sprinkle each serving with cilantro.

❧ TOFU SALAD ☙

(Serves at least 4)

Tofu Salad is terrific served hot with rice for a family dinner or it can be refrigerated and used throughout the week for lunches and snacks.

1 cake firm tofu
2 freshly scrubbed carrots
2 cloves garlic finely minced
3 tablespoons olive oil
1/4 teaspoon turmeric
1/4 teaspoon minced ginger
Pinch coriander
2 tablespoons lemon juice
1 to 1 1/2 tablespoons tamari
2 stalks chopped celery

Optional:
Handful chopped parsley
1/4 cup sunflower seeds
Several chopped green onions

1. Grate carrots by hand, or with a food processor, into a large mixing bowl. Drain tofu and mix in with carrots mashing with a potato masher, a pastry cutter or your hands.

2. In a separate container mix together lemon juice, tamari, garlic, and spices.

3. Heat olive oil in a large deep skillet on medium-high heat. Stir carrot tofu mixture into olive oil until well mixed. Cover, and allow to cook 2 to 3 minutes.

4. Add chopped celery and sauté a minute more.

5. Stir in spice mixture. Add any or all of the optional items and adjust tamari to taste. Refrigerated this dish can last 5 days.

✎ CHILEAN PINTOS ✎

2 cups dried pinto beans, rinsed and soaked overnight
    in 3 cups of pure or filtered water
1 (10 oz.) bag of frozen organic corn or one ear fresh corn
    removed from the cob
2 teaspoons sesame oil
1 onion, chopped

Garnish:
3 cloves garlic
Minced chopped green onion
1 teaspoon dried oregano
Squeeze of fresh lemon
½ teaspoon sea salt
Chopped cilantro

1. Place beans and soaking water in a large pot. Add 1 cup more pure or filtered water to cover. Cover pot and bring to a boil, reduce heat and simmer, stirring occasionally, for 1 to ½ hours until beans are almost tender.

2. Heat sesame oil in a medium skillet. Sauté onions until almost translucent. Add garlic, oregano, and salt and sauté a few minutes longer. Add corn and stir well into onion mixture until thoroughly defrosted. Using a heat-resistant rubber spatula scrape onion-corn mixture into the beans stirring in well.

Cook over medium heat stirring frequently for about
10 more minutes.

3. Serve in large bowls over rice or other favorite grain.
Garnish generously.

⤳ SOUTHERN BLACK-EYED PEAS ⤳

If you're lucky you may find fresh black-eyed peas in the pod at your
local farmer's market. A little extra work shucking these peas will
give you a delicate and flavorful treat. This dish is still wonderful
with the dried variety however.

> 1 cup fresh or dried black-eyed peas, soaked overnight
> 2 cup pure or filtered water
> 1 ½ teaspoons sea salt
> 1 tablespoon butter
> 1 onion
> 3 cloves garlic
> ¼ teaspoon allspice
> Pinch cayenne (optional)
> Tamari to taste
> Optional garnish: chopped tomato, chopped parsley

1. Drain black-eyed peas and discard soaking water. Place peas,
   water and salt into a medium saucepan. Bring to a boil, cover,
   and reduce heat to simmer ½ hour.

2. Meanwhile chop onion and mince garlic. When peas are almost
   tender melt butter in a large skillet. Add onion and garlic and
   sauté on medium until onion becomes translucent but not
   browned. Stir in allspice and cayenne, if using. Pour cooked
   peas and cooking water into onion-spice mixture. Stir well and
   allow to simmer 10 minutes uncovered. Season generously
   with tamari to taste. Serve over brown rice with a sprinkling of
   tomato or parsley if you'd like.

❧ WHITE BEANS WITH SAGE ❧

A gourmet dish, this recipe is inspired by a similar one in *Fields of Greens,* a terrific gourmet vegetarian manual. Use fresh sage, if available, but the dried variety is also delicious. Serve over brown rice.

> 2 cans or 4 cups cooked organic navy, great northern, or other white beans with liquid
> 1 cup pure or filtered water
> 2 bay leaves
> 1 teaspoon dried sage, plus 1/4 teaspoon or 5 leaves of fresh sage, chopped
> ½ teaspoon dried thyme
> 3 tablespoons olive oil
> 1 onion
> 3 cloves garlic
> Sea salt to taste
> Tamari to taste
> Large handful of chopped parsley (Italian is nice)
> Wine to taste (optional)

1. Place beans, water, bay leaves, thyme, and 1 teaspoon dried or 3 leaves fresh sage in a medium saucepan. Bring to a low simmer and cook for 10 minutes.

2. Meanwhile chop onion and mince garlic.

3. Heat olive oil in a large skillet on medium heat. Add onion and a few pinches of salt. Sauté about five minutes until onions become slightly translucent. Add garlic and the remaining sage and sauté a few minutes more. Add wine, if using, and cook, stirring frequently, until the pan is nearly dry.

4. Add the beans to the onion mixture along with ½ teaspoon salt. Cover and cook for 15 to 20 minutes on low. Stir in a few dashes of tamari to taste. Just before serving stir in the chopped parsley.

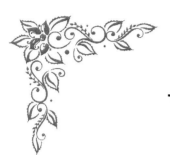

15

Vegetables

Cooking Vegetables

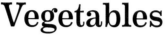

e buy fresh, organically grown vegetables whenever possible. Get to know your local food co-ops, farmer's markets, and health food stores. Farmer's markets can be the best places to purchase low cost organic produce. Vegetables will be fresher when purchased directly from the farmer. Many vendors in these markets pick their produce the same day they bring it to market. If you can, use these fruits and vegetables as soon as you get home from the market. You will taste the difference.

Buy vegetables when they are in season to assure freshness and taste. Corn in January, unless you live in the tropics, will be a long way from the plant that grew it and probably fairly tasteless. Buy a vegetable for its looks and smell rather than buying for a recipe. A recipe can't tell you what vegetables will be fresh and in season in the market. When you see a great deal on some gorgeous looking English peas, for instance, take them home and figure out how to cook them.

The following guide discusses the vegetables that will be most beneficial to your diet. This alphabetical index will explain how to shop for and prepare vegetables. We've also included some of our favorite vegetable recipes. Some vegetables will be familiar and others you may never have cooked with before. We recommend you try as many as you can find in the store. It's almost impossible for the average person to eat too many vegetables.

Steaming Vegetables

Steaming is one of the best methods for cooking vegetables. Done correctly, steaming brings out and preserves the vegetables' vitamins and beauty.

Use high-quality "waterless" cookware made of stainless steel or enamel coating. Do not use aluminum cookware. A tight fitting lid is essential for waterless cooking. Waterless means that the lid should seal itself during the steaming process.

Add just enough water to the pot to barely cover the bottom. Add 1 teaspoon oil, (olive, coconut, sesame, or other favorite), or butter. Place chopped vegetables into pot and cover. Heat pot on a medium-high flame until filled with steam.

You may need to reduce heat if the pressure of the steam is too high and steam is streaming out from under the lid. Steam vegetables just until they are tender and at the height of their color. This can be from 1 minute, such as for spinach, or up to 15 minutes or more for tougher vegetables such as carrots.

Steaming is not an exact science. It is difficult to give an exact time for cooking steamed vegetables. There are too many variables such as vegetable size, steam temperature, etc. You must monitor your vegetables closely to assure they do not overcook. But, avoid lifting the cover too much or most of the steam will escape along with precious vitamins. If you must err in cooking, undercook rather than overcook your vegetables. Often vegetables taste delicious when steamed only briefly and they are still crispy.

It won't take long to become an expert at steaming your favorite vegetables. Once you have the knack, it will be hard to understand how you ever lived without this skill before.

ARTICHOKES

Buy artichokes that are bright green with tight buds. At home, submerge the artichokes in cold water and swish around to remove any dirt or bugs hidden in the leaves.

Fresh artichokes are simple to prepare. Trim the stem and remove any small, outer leaves from it leaving a nice tight bud. Place the artichokes with the stems down in an airtight pot in about half an inch of water. Steam 20 to 30 minutes, depending on size, until a fork inserted into the base of the stem slides in easily. (Artichokes, unlike most vegetables, cannot be eaten at the height of its color. It must be cooked beyond this point to be edible.)

To eat, pull leaves off flower one at a time. Dip meaty heart end into a little melted lemon butter and using your teeth scrape meat off end of leaf. Repeat until you've reached the hairy inside of the artichoke. Using a spoon scrape the inedible hairs out of the heart being careful not to scrape out the meat with the hairs. The delicious heart of the artichoke is your reward for your diligence. Dip into the lemon butter and eat down to the base of the stem. The flavor is unlike any canned artichoke heart you will ever find.

ARUGULA

Arugula has a strong spicy smell. Younger leaves, smaller and more delicate, tend to be stronger in flavor. These small leaves are what gourmets tend to look for. However, larger leaves are still delicious and, for new arugula eaters, can be strong enough.

Arugula makes an exotic salad. Try tossing leaves with olive oil, orange juice and a pinch of salt. Add carefully peeled orange chunks or sliced kumquats. Mix arugula with leafy lettuce if you want to cut its bite.

ASPARAGUS

Asparagus is an elegant green vegetable and one of the easiest to cook. Prepare asparagus by rinsing and trimming off the bottom inch of the stems. This part is woody and unpleasant to chew. Steam whole asparagus laid flat in a large sauté pan with an airtight lid. Fresh asparagus will take only a minute or two to reach a vivid green. Under cooking asparagus slightly will leave it crunchy and delicious. Wonderful with lemon butter with just a hint of lemon zest. Also, you can cut the asparagus and stir-fry it.

AVOCADO

We use avocados as often as we can get them. Cut up for salads there is no equal. Avocados are also great on toast for a quick snack. I like to spread a few slices onto a nice grainy bread and squeeze a little lemon on top. Top with sesame salt for a real treat.

Avocados will turn brown in the refrigerator with their seed. Cut the avocado from around its seed and store in plastic to prevent the flesh from browning. The exposed edges will brown but the meat will stay green and delicious. This trick of laying plastic wrap on top will keep avocado dip from turning brown as well.

BEETS

Beets are a super-nutritious vegetable. We recommend you eat them frequently. Too often the delicious and nutritious greens of the beet are thrown away. These greens are wonderful steamed or sautéed alone, or throw them in with your favorite beetroot recipe. It's not necessary to peel beets; just scrub them firmly with the scouring side of a sponge until hairs and dirt are removed.

❧ HOT BEET SALAD ❧

(Serves 4 generously)

2 tablespoons sesame seeds
3 medium beets with tops
1 tablespoon sesame oil
1 tablespoon lemon juice
1 tablespoon tamari

1. Rinse sesame seeds in strainer and place in a large skillet (no oil) on medium-high heat until water evaporates. Turn heat to low and toast a minute or two until seeds are fragrant. Stir or shake skillet once or twice to brown evenly. Set aside.

2. Scrub the roots of the beets, trim off the tail, and peel the dirty part of the root below the stems. Swish the beet tops in a sink full of water to remove dirt. Grate the roots in a food processor or by hand. Chop the beet leaves coarsely and set aside.

3. In a large skillet or wok heat sesame oil over medium-high heat. When hot add beet roots, leaves and stems and cook stirring frequently for about 10 minutes until beet roots are crispy and leaves are wilted. Add lemon juice, tamari and sesame seeds. Stir and serve.

BROCCOLI

Broccoli is known for its nutritive value but, many people have only experienced overcooked or frozen broccoli and don't know its wonderful flavor. As with most vegetables, broccoli should only be cooked to the height of its color. Once its green brightness starts fading, broccoli's nutritive value and taste quickly plummet.

To cook broccoli, wash thoroughly in cold water. (Broccoli is one of those blessed green vegetables that grow far above the ground and do not need much more than a quick rinse to clean.) Trim about an inch off the stem ends. Using a sharp knife, peel broccoli stems. Start at the stem end, inserting the knife under the fibrous peel. Grasp the peel between the knife and thumb and rip up and off the stem. Keep leaves and flowerets that get removed along with stem. You don't have to be a perfect stem peeler; however, make sure that the bottom part of the stem, where the peel is the toughest, is peel free. Cut the stem into ½-inch thick rounds, or into sticks if you prefer. Separate broccoli head into flowerets. Steam broccoli all at once. Season with tamari-lemon butter.

BRUSSELS SPROUTS

Unfortunately, these broccoli relatives have a terrible reputation among most people. They are quite healthy, but also delicious when steamed to perfection, salted, and popped in the mouth. Remove browned leaves from Brussels sprouts and trim the stems. Steamed Brussels sprouts are done when a fork can easily slide into the center. Do not overcook Brussels sprouts or they will acquire their famous bitterness. Try the following recipe.

✎ KIDS-LOVE-EM BRUSSELS SPROUTS ✎

Anyone will love Brussels sprouts cooked this way, not just kids. Try substituting carrots, or spinach, or any other vegetable you're having a hard time convincing someone, or yourself, to eat.

1 lb. Brussels sprouts
3 tablespoons butter
2 tablespoons maple syrup
Salt to taste

1. Wash and trim Brussels sprouts removing any browned outside leaves.

2. In a large sauté pan with a lid, melt 1 tablespoon of the butter over low heat. Stir in Brussels sprouts coating them with the

butter. Increase heat to medium, cover, and allow to cook 10 minutes until sprouts are bright green and a fork slides in easily when poked.

3. Meanwhile, in a small saucepan or in the microwave, melt the 2 remaining tablespoons of butter with the maple syrup. Pour over the Brussels sprouts and serve.

CABBAGE

Cabbage is quite high in Vitamin C and is good juiced. It lacks the high Vitamin A of other leafy vegetables so it's not recommended as a frequent part of your diet. However, cabbage is wonderful combined with other vegetables in a stir-fry or a soup. Here, its subtle flavor shines.

◈ PURPLE CABBAGE AND CELERY SLAW ◈

This is a pretty and tasty salad.

3 stalks celery
½ head purple cabbage
1 tablespoon lemon juice
1 tablespoon unrefined sesame oil
¼ teaspoon salt
2 tablespoons sunflower seeds

Chop celery and shred cabbage into small bite-size pieces. Toss together all ingredients.

CARROTS

Carrots are another vegetable we always have on hand. Famous for their high content of Vitamin A, carrots are not overrated. Carrots are the vegetable one finds hidden in the vegetable crisper drawer when everything else has been eaten. They make a wonderful side dish simply steamed and tossed with butter and parsley, (another back of the refrigerator herb.) Try serving sliced and steamed beets and carrots together. Be sure to steam the vegetables separately to attain the pretty marbling of orange and red when the carrots and beets are finally tossed together. Toss with a little olive oil and lemon for a beautiful dish. Carrots are also essential to juicing.

A steady and inexpensive supply of bulk organic carrots is a necessity to any serious juicer owner. Carrot juice adds palatability and vitamin content to other vegetable juices. Do not drink it by itself, as its sugar content is too high for many people. You will find that organic carrots are inexpensive bought in bulk and they keep for weeks in the refrigerator. Bulk carrots are a basic addition to any soup or stir-fry. More expensive are the fresher carrots that are often sold with their green tops still attached. These carrots are often sweeter and better for salads or just munching as is. Save the green tops in the freezer for soup stock. Try this sweet, festive carrot recipe.

ᑐᕈ CARROTS WITH MAPLE-PECAN GLAZE ᕈᑐ

3 large carrots
½ cup pecan halves or pieces
2 teaspoons butter
1 tablespoon maple syrup
¼ cup orange juice
½ teaspoon sea salt

1. Chop carrots neatly into rounds. Steam in 1 tablespoon of water with 1 teaspoon of the butter for about 10 minutes or until softened but still crisp.

2. In a separate skillet, toast the pecans over medium heat stirring occasionally until evenly browned and fragrant. Add remaining butter, maple syrup, and orange juice. When butter has melted stir in carrots and cook, stirring frequently, until orange juice is reduced to a glaze, about 10 minutes.

CAULIFLOWER

Cauliflower makes a wonderful soup and is great added to a stir-fry. However, cauliflower is lacking in the vitamin A that most people need from vegetables. Try substituting broccoli flower, a hybrid of cauliflower and broccoli, in recipes that call for cauliflower. Broccoli flower with Yogurt-Curry sauce is a delicious treat.

CELERY

Celery is a staple for soup stock and stuffing. We always have celery in our refrigerator. It keeps a long time and is great for filling out a soup or stir-fry recipe. Sautéed with garlic and onions, celery is a great beginning to any dish.

CORN

In the summer corn is an irresistible treat. Corn bought at the height of the season will be sweet and large with healthy husks. Try eating corn as soon a you buy it. The longer uncooked corn spends off the plant the more its sugars turn to starches and vitamins are lost. Fresh corn on the cob does not have the starch content of corn-meal or popcorn, so it is okay to eat on your diet.

The best way to cook fresh corn is to slow grill it in the husks. Cover the threaded ends of the ear with a little aluminum foil to prevent burning and place ears over a hot grill, turning occasionally until done, usually about 20 to 30 minutes, or you can cook corn in a 400°F oven in the husk for 30 to 40 minutes.

Many people boil corn but the loss of vitamins and sugars with this method can leave the corn fairly tasteless. When eating corn on the cob, be sure to eat the germ of the corn. The germ is the smaller pieces under the kernels often left uneaten by ravenous corn eaters. The germ is the most nutritious part however, so be sure to eat it all.

Frozen, organic corn is a good option when fresh corn isn't in season. Frozen corn retains much of its sugars and vitamins when frozen quickly after being picked. Thus, frozen corn is a better option than older, "fresh" corn. We like to add frozen corn to our soups and stews.

GREENS

Dark leafy greens are among the most nutritious vegetables we can eat. There are an endless variety of greens in the world. Here is a list, certainly not complete, of those most readily available: kale, collard, chard, escarole, mustard, beet, watercress, arugula, spinach, bok choy, rapini, Chinese broccoli, dandelion, and turnip.

Use fresh greens with crisp leaves that aren't wilted or yellowed. Greens such as spinach will need to be washed thoroughly to remove dirt and grit, or you can buy pre-washed greens. Make sure pre-washed greens are fresh before purchasing. To wash greens submerge them in a sink full of cold water and swish them around allowing dirt to sink to bottom of sink. If greens are especially dirty, repeat. Greens such as kale and mustards will need to be removed from the stem before cooking, as the stems are too tough to eat. Generally, greens should be chopped or torn into bite-size pieces before cooking.

Collard greens are cheap and delicious and not just for Southerners anymore. Buy the dark green leaves while they are crispy and cook them soon after purchasing. Wilted or old leaves are often tough and lack the vitamin and calcium kick of freshly picked leaves. Steam or sauté collards as you would other leafy greens. Avoid overcooking them. Traditionally, collards are served with a dash of vinegar but try substituting lemon juice and butter.

Raddichio is commonly used in gourmet salad mix. However, raddichio is wonderful sautéed with escarole or spinach. Try combining these greens and lightly sautéing in olive oil with red onion and a squeeze of lemon. Serve on whole grain toast as a healthier version of Bruschetta.

⸎ THAI-STYLE STIR-FRIED GREENS ⸎

This recipe is a great way to experiment with new varieties of greens. Make this dish into a meal by combining with fried tofu and serving with rice. If you desire, substitute a few teaspoons Thai fish sauce for the tamari for an authentic Thai side dish.

2 teaspoons coconut oil
2 cloves garlic, minced
¼ teaspoon crushed red chili
1 bunch fresh greens
2 teaspoons tamari, plus more to taste
1 teaspoon toasted sesame oil

1. Thoroughly wash greens by submerging in water and swishing to remove dirt. Remove any wilted or yellowed leaves. Remove any tough parts such as the spine of the kale or collard leaves. You may want to peel the stems of Chinese broccoli to make them tender. Coarsely chop greens and have ready before beginning to stir-fry.

2. Heat sesame oil in a large skillet or wok on medium high. Add garlic and red chili and cook stirring constantly for 30 seconds but don't let garlic burn. Add greens and stir leaves into the hot oil. Leaves will reduce in size quickly. Add tamari and continue to stir greens until they've reached the brightest green. Stir in toasted sesame oil and quickly remove from pan. Serve immediately.

GREEN BEANS

A wonderfully versatile vegetable, green beans are at the height of their season in the summer. Steam green beans until bright green and toss with butter, lemon, and a little fresh or dried dill for a heavenly summer treat. Green beans are also a wonderful addition to a stir-fry and can be added when you add the broccoli spears.

Try sautéing green beans with yellow squash, onions, and garlic. Season with tamari and toss with pasta.

Choose crispy beans that snap easily when broken in two. To prepare green beans simply rinse and snap or trim off the stem end. The tail does not need trimming. For fast trimming lay a dozen or more green beans on a cutting board with the stems lined up. Use a sharp knife to trim all the stem ends at once.

This is an elegant recipe with many variations. Add lemon juice, tamari and herbs to taste.

❧ GREEN BEANS WITH BASIL ☙

1 lb. green beans, (or any fresh summer beans)
1 tablespoon olive oil
2 cloves garlic, minced
2 tablespoons lemon juice
¼ teaspoon sea salt
Handful of fresh basil, chopped, (or substitute fresh dill)
Tamari to taste
Wine to taste (optional)

1. Place a medium pot of lightly salted water on high heat and bring to a boil. Meanwhile, rinse and trim the inedible stem part off the green beans. When water has boiled drop the beans in the water and allow to parboil 2 to 3 minutes or just until their colors reach their brightest. Drain and rinse well with cold water to keep beans from continuing to cook.

2. Heat olive oil in a large skillet on medium. Add garlic, lemon juice, and wine. Cook, stirring frequently, until liquids are significantly reduced, about 3 minutes. Add the beans, salt, and basil and continue to stir and sauté for a few minutes more until beans are warmed and basil is slightly wilted but still bright green. Dash with a little tamari to taste and serve immediately.

RADISHES

Radishes aren't just for salads but can be a beautiful way to add to a stir-fry or steamed vegetable mixture. When cooked the pepper of the radish mellows to a succulent flavor.

One of the healthiest radishes around is the Daikon radish, which is common to Asian cooking. Daikon is wonderful in Miso soup or raw and thinly sliced into a salad. They are sweeter than the domestic varieties of radish so many prefer them.

PARSNIPS

Parsnips are often overlooked in American diets, but any connoisseur of chicken soup knows they are an essential ingredient. Parsnips should never be boiled in water because they are quite sweet, and the water dissolves out the sugar, leaving mush! Scrub and scrape if necessary, slice thin, and stir-fry, bake, or add to soups. Parsnips add a wonderful sweet flavor to soup stocks and can be cooked and used the same way one would potatoes. Grilled parsnips sliced open and spread with a pat of butter are absolutely delicious.

PEAS

Peas are one of those few vegetables that almost everyone gets along with. If you can find fresh English peas in the summer you will have a taste sensation that you won't find in frozen peas. Shell

English peas and steam or sauté them and eat them immediately. They hardly need seasoning. They make a wonderful addition to a salad. Try making a faux Nicoise salad with tuna and English peas on a bed of lettuce with a light homemade mayonnaise dressing.

Frozen peas are often more nutritious than fresh. The peas are frozen immediately after picking so they retain their vitamins and color, which can fade quickly. Frozen peas are also useful as a quick addition to Miso soup, salads, pasta, or just frozen straight out of the bag. Kids love frozen peas.

Snow peas are common additions to stir-fry and are also wonderful raw in salads. Buy fresh, wash, and simply snap off the stem end.

SHIITAKE MUSHROOMS

A staple of macrobiotic diet these are the only mushrooms people with severe Candida should eat. Fresh shiitake mushrooms are sometimes available in health food stores and are a wonderful addition to a sauté. The dried variety are more readily available in the macrobiotic section of your health food store. They add a nice, mellow flavor to soup. Just be sure to soak the mushrooms to reconstitute them, (add the soaking water to the soup as well,) and remove the inedible stems. To soak, place mushrooms stem-side down in a large bowl and pour warm water over. Allow to soak 30 minutes, drain, and cut the mushrooms down to the appropriate size. Reserve the soaking water for soup stock.

SPROUTS

Nowadays, there is endless variety in the types of sprouts available. Happily, we are no longer stuck with plain alfalfa sprouts. Sprouts can give an extra crunch to almost any dish. Sunflower sprouts are wonderful on sandwiches, and bean sprouts are delicious in miso soup or other Asian-style fare. Also available in health food stores are sprouted, mixed legumes. They are a healthful addition to soups or stir-fry. Sprouts provide a high concentration of detoxifying enzymes, but do not contain as much vitamin A, vitamin C, and minerals as mature, green, leafy vegetables.

SUMMER SQUASH

Zucchini, crookneck, yellow and other summer squashes are true flags of summer. Buy them at the market and bring them home with a bunch of fresh basil to sauté as light side dish. Try a sauté of summer squash, Italian herbs, and onions and garlic over whole grain pasta.

TURNIPS

Freshly picked turnips with the greens still attached are a real treat. Cut the roots into bite-sized chunks and steam. In the last few minutes of steaming add the chopped turnip greens. Toss with butter and salt and enjoy.

Turnips are also wonderful added to soups and sautés. Try a side dish of steamed turnips, radishes, parsnips, and carrots, adding a little garlic sautéed in butter and/or olive oil; or roast the roots in a 325°F oven, basting frequently with garlic infused olive oil.

WINTER SQUASH

Prick a whole winter squash with a fork several times all over and place in a baking dish. Bake at 350°F until a fork slides into squash easily. When done, slice open squash while still hot and remove seeds, slather on a little butter and salt and eat straight out of the skin. Be sure to try the Winter Squash Soup in the soups section.

16

Salads and Dressings

Salad Greens

rganic salad mixes, such as mesclun, are sold in most health food stores nowadays. Recently, there has been a surge of interest in exotic salad greens. The varieties you will find, even if you live outside of California, offer plenty of salad experimenting. Try any or all of the greens on this list plus any others you find in your local market: arugula, endive, hearts of escarole, frisee, raddichio, red or green bibb lettuce, red or green leaf lettuce, romaine, and watercress.

Wash salad greens well, especially spinach, which is notoriously muddy. Submerge the greens in a sink full of water and gently swish allowing dirt to fall to sink bottom. Repeat until no dirt settles to the bottom of the sink. Spin dry in a salad spinner, a must for a flavorful salad without watered down dressing. If you don't have a salad spinner gently pat greens dry in a clean cloth towel.

Consider, also, leafy greens that aren't traditionally used for salad. Baby beet leaves, pale, young dandelion leaves, and thin slices of sorrel are all wonderful ways to fill out and heighten the flavor of a salad. Other wonderful additions to salads are fresh, seasonal herbs. A few delicately torn leaves of fresh basil, fresh oregano, or sprigs of dill make a salad a masterpiece. Try adding fruits and nuts such as apples with toasted walnuts or oranges with toasted pecans in an orange-lemon dressing. A wonderful and exotic combination is Asian pears with purple basil. Experiment with additions of your own. Make the salad a meal by adding beans or grains. Salads are also a wonderful way to use up leftovers. There are few food items you can't put into a salad. These additions can turn your salads into exciting gourmet dishes! Forget those boring iceberg lettuce salads. Iceberg lettuce has little or no vitamin A or Cup

Salad dressings should be where you use your best ingredients. Use the freshest, juiciest lemons and the finest, cold-pressed organic olive oil or other oil. Keep homemade salad dressing handy in the refrigerator. For a quick meal you can pull out some prewashed mesclun salad mix, throw in leftover beans and rice or leftover toasted nuts, some avocado, toss with oil and dressing and voila!

⤳ INCREDIBLE SALAD DRESSING ⤶

If you are using dried herbs this dressing can be kept in a tightly closed container in the refrigerator for up to a week. In fact, like a good soup this dressing tastes even better after a few days. Dressings made with fresh herbs need to be used the same day.

2 tablespoons fresh lemon juice (approximately 1 lemon)
1 to 2 cloves pressed or minced garlic (to taste)
Pinch of any or all of the following herbs: (dried or freshly chopped) thyme, marjoram, rosemary, basil, and dill
(My favorite combination is marjoram, dill, and thyme.)
1 tablespoon tamari (or more to taste)

1. Mix above ingredients and allow to stand at least five minutes while flavors blend.

2. Toss 2 tablespoons olive oil or pumpkin seed oil with 4 to 6 cups of mixed greens. Add lemon juice mixture and toss again. Add any other vegetables you'd like such as tomatoes, cucumbers, or avocados. Add wet ingredients, such as tomatoes, just before serving salad. Enjoy!

ORANGE DRESSING

This dressing is best used fresh.

Zest of half an organic orange (about 1 teaspoon)
2 tablespoons orange juice
1 tablespoon lemon juice
¼ teaspoon sea salt
3 tablespoons olive oil

1. Using a sharp knife peel the orange part from the outside of a washed orange avoiding the bitter white pith. Use the knife to scrape away any white pith that may remain on your peelings. This is the zest of the orange. Slice the zest into thin strips.

2. Combine all ingredients except the olive oil. Whisk in olive oil and pour over an exotic salad of baby greens, orange pieces, and toasted nuts.

TAHINI DRESSING

(Makes about 1 cup)

This Middle Eastern staple can be watered down slightly to make a great salad dressing. Or use it thick for a protein-rich sauce to drizzle over vegetables or grains.

½ cup tahini
Juice of 1 large lemon, (about 4 tablespoons)
2 cloves garlic, pressed
½ cup water
¼ teaspoon sea salt

Mix tahini and lemon juice well until there are no lumps. Stir in garlic. Add water a little at a time blending well. Thin with more water as desired. Stir in sea salt and serve.

HOMEMADE MAYONNAISE

1 egg*
1/2 teaspoon sea salt
1/2 teaspoon mustard powder (dry)
2 tablespoons lemon juice
1 cup olive oil (Omega Nutrition preferred)

Place egg, sea salt, mustard powder, and lemon juice in blender or food processor. Slowly, in a thin, steady stream, pour olive oil into blender or food processor while blending on low.

*Note: This must be a fertile egg from a free-range chicken, and must be quite fresh. Do not use regular grocery store eggs. They are lacking in nutritional value, and they can give you a salmonella infection.

DILLED AVOCADO SALAD

This salad works well in pita bread or wrapped in a tortilla. The cheese is a nice addition but not necessary to make this a satisfying side dish or snack.

1 avocado, cubed
1 cucumber, halved, seeded and sliced thin
1/2 red pepper, cubed small (optional)
1 green onion, chopped
2 tablespoons fresh dill, chopped
1 tablespoon olive oil
Juice of half a lemon
1/2 cup mild & firm white cheese, cubed (optional)

Combine all ingredients and gently toss.

YOGURT-CUCUMBER SALAD

2 tablespoons minced fresh dill
2 cloves garlic, pressed
1 1/2 cup plain yogurt
1 large cucumber peeled and thinly sliced

Combine dill, garlic and yogurt. Add cucumber and combine thoroughly. Serve or refrigerate immediately.

VARIATION: Substitute 1/4 teaspoon ground cumin for the dill.

FRUIT SALAD

Slice 3 to 4 cups of fruit from the following list:

Papaya
Banana
Strawberries
Kiwi
Pear
Blueberries
Raspberries

Mix in large bowl with the juice of 1 lime and a small bunch of fresh chopped mint leaves. To sweeten salad, add 1 tablespoon maple syrup or more to taste.

17

Seasonings

Without seasonings in our food, a meal is a dull venture. The recipes in this book have suggested seasonings for each dish. If they are not according to your taste, experiment within the following guidelines.

Salt is necessary for many dishes to enhance the flavor, but do not use salt to excess, especially if you are trying to bring down your blood pressure. Never use salt with chemical additives. Some of them can be toxic. For seasoning your food after cooking, I suggest you stick to the following salty seasonings:

Miso: a salty soybean paste that can be diluted with water and added to vegetables, grains and soups.

Tamari: similar to miso, but liquid, so it can be sprinkled on food.

Sesame salt: which is low in sodium but tastes quite salty (see recipe).

Ume plum paste: quite salty and quite sour. This is an acquired taste for most people, so start off with a small amount. I find it exquisite on corn on the cob.

Red pepper: can be quite irritating to some people, but, if you can tolerate it, it stimulates circulation and can help in detoxifying the body. The best rule is to avoid it for the first few weeks of your program and then try it in moderation.

You can use any fresh herbs in moderation. Do not use strong spices until you are fairly far along in your program.

Do not use black pepper. It is an irritant to the digestive tract. White pepper is from the same plant and should be avoided, also.

HOW TO MAKE SESAME SALT

Use sesame salt on everything instead of salt. It can even make plain brown rice a delicious snack. Sesame salt is best if made fresh every week.

1 1/2 teaspoon sea salt
1/2 cup unhulled sesame seeds

1. Wash the sesame seeds well in pure water; use a strainer; drain.

2. Roast the salt in a large cast iron or stainless steel skillet for about five minutes over medium heat. Pour the salt into your food processor.

3. Turn the heat down under the skillet to low. Add the sesame seeds and stir constantly until seeds are dry and begin to toast. Note: if the heat is too high the sesame seeds will pop like popcorn. Allow to toast a few minutes until seeds become fragrant, darken in color, and burst open when a few of them are pinched between the fingers.

4. Add the seeds to the food processor. Grind the salt and seeds together for 60 seconds or until a majority of the seeds are no longer whole.

5. Store in an airtight jar and use instead of regular salt. You can also store sesame salt in the freezer in an airtight jar or bag. Allow bag to come to room temperature before opening to keep moisture out.

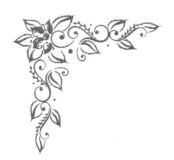

18

Sweets

APPLESAUCE PAN CAKE

2 beaten eggs
2 tablespoons sesame or almond oil (Omega Nutrition
   preferred)
1 cup applesauce
½ cup almond milk, organic milk, or pure or filtered water
½ cup maple syrup
½ teaspoon cinnamon
¼ teaspoon nutmeg
¼ teaspoon grated ginger
2 cups whole grain pancake mix
1 tablespoon coconut oil or butter

1. Blend eggs, oil, applesauce, liquid, maple syrup, cinnamon, nutmeg, and ginger. Stir in pancake mix. Heat coconut oil or butter in an 8-inch skillet. Pour in batter and heat on medium flame until edges start to look done.

2. Bake in 350°F oven until center is done (knife inserted in center is not wet with dough; approximately 20 minutes).

MAPLE PECAN MUFFINS

(Makes 18 muffins)

These muffins will stay fresh for several days if stored in an airtight container in the refrigerator. A high-energy snack, they also make a delicious and quick breakfast.

1 ½ cup maple syrup

3 eggs, separated (see Separating Eggs below*)

3 tablespoons melted butter

2 cup whole-wheat pasty flour

½ teaspoon sea salt

1 ½ teaspoons baking powder

¼ teaspoon each cinnamon, nutmeg, allspice

2 cups (8 oz.) raw pecans, chopped

1. Preheat oven to 350°F.

2. Butter muffin tins or line with paper muffin cups. Whisk yolks with maple syrup and butter in a large mixing bowl.

3. Measure flour, salt, baking powder and spices into sifter and sift directly into maple syrup mixture. Combine just until mixture is fairly uniform.

4. In a separate bowl, beat egg yolks with an electric mixer on high until stiff peaks form. Using a rubber spatula, fold egg whites into batter until just incorporated. Don't worry if egg whites are not thoroughly combined.

5. Add chopped pecans to mix reserving about ¼ cup to sprinkle on top of muffins. Avoid over stirring.

6. Fill muffin tins about ⅔ full. Sprinkle with chopped pecans and bake 20 minutes until knife inserted into the center of a muffin comes out clean.

* To separate eggs have two bowls ready. Crack egg on edge of bowl neatly in the middle. Holding shell halves close together slowly pour yolk back and forth from one half of shell to other allowing the whites to drain into bowl underneath. Pour yolk into separate bowl. This may take some practice. Be careful not to get any yolk in with the whites as whites won't beat well with yolk in them.

❧ WHEAT GERM BLONDIES ❧

2 eggs
¼ cup almond oil, sesame oil or melted butter
¾ cup maple syrup
1 teaspoon vanilla
2 cups wheat germ
½ cup barley flour
½ teaspoon non-aluminum baking powder
½ cup broken walnuts or pecans

1. Line the bottom of an 8 x 8-inch baking dish with wax paper. You'll have to use scissors to make it fit. Grease the wax paper and sides of dish with butter or oil.

2. Preheat oven to 350°F.

3. Use a whisk or fork to beat the eggs in large mixing bowl. Beat in oil or melted butter, maple syrup and vanilla. In a separate bowl mix dry ingredients to distribute baking powder then add to wet ingredients. Mix in nuts.

4. Spread batter evenly in dish and bake for 30 minutes.

5. When done slide a knife around the edges and turn immediately out of dish. Remove wax paper and cut into squares while hot. Wheat Germ Blondies are best eaten chilled.

❧ ALMOND BUTTER COOKIES ❧

½ cup butter, softened
1 ½ cup almond butter
1 ½ cup maple syrup
2 ½ cup whole-wheat pastry flour
½ teaspoon sea salt
¼ teaspoon cinnamon
35 to 40 raw, whole almonds (optional)

1. Preheat oven to 325°F.

2. Stir butter into almond butter with a fork or an electric mixer. Add maple syrup in stages until well mixed.

3. Combine flour, salt and cinnamon in a separate bowl. Add to the wet ingredients and mix well until flour is thoroughly moistened.

4. Drop teaspoonfuls of dough onto a lightly buttered cookie sheet spacing them at least one inch apart. Flatten cookies slightly with a fork dipped in flour or press a whole almond into the center of each cookie.

5. Bake 25 to 30 minutes. Cool slightly on cookie sheet before removing or they will fall apart.

⋘ SQUASH COOKIES ⋙

These cookies are moist and chewy and quite satisfying.

6 tablespoons butter, allowed to soften
2 cup cooked winter squash
3/4 cup maple syrup
1/2 teaspoon vanilla extract
2 cup barley flour
1 1/2 teaspoons baking powder
1/4 teaspoon sea salt
1/4 teaspoon cinnamon
1/4 teaspoon powdered cardamom (optional)
1/2 cup chopped walnuts (optional)

1. Preheat oven to 350°F.

2. In a large mixing bowl cream softened butter and squash together until thoroughly mixed. (You may use a food processor but it's not necessary unless you are using stringy squash.) Mix in maple syrup and vanilla.

3. In a separate bowl, combine flour, baking powder, salt and spices.

4. Add dry ingredients to wet ingredients stirring well. A rubber spatula works well here.

5. Lightly butter a cookie sheet. Drop heaping spoonfuls of batter at least an inch apart on cookie sheet. Flatten batter with spoon or your fingers. Bake 25 minutes or until cookies are lightly browned on the bottom.

❧ PEACH CAKE ☙

2 cup whole-wheat pastry flour
¾ teaspoon baking soda
½ teaspoon salt
½ teaspoon cinnamon
¼ teaspoon allspice
2 eggs
1 cup maple syrup
½ cup plain or vanilla yogurt
1 teaspoon vanilla extract
¼ teaspoon almond extract
2 tablespoons melted butter
2 to 3 cup sliced peaches, fresh or frozen and defrosted

1. Preheat oven to 350°F.

2. Generously butter a 9 x 13 baking pan. Sift together flour, baking soda, salt, and spices into a large mixing bowl.

3. In a separate bowl beat the eggs together. Add maple syrup, yogurt, vanilla and almond extracts, and finally butter, stirring between each addition.

4. Pour wet ingredients into dry stirring as you pour to mix. Mix only until flour is moistened. Gently fold in peaches using a rubber spatula.

5. Pour batter into a baking pan and gently spread to edges. Bake for 30 minutes or until a knife inserted in cake comes out clean.

6. Serve hot or cold with a dollop of maple yogurt. Try mixing yogurt with 1 teaspoon of rum or ¼ teaspoon almond extract.

❧ POUND CAKE ❧

This pound cake is a long way from the rich old-fashioned cake, which required 1 pound each of flour, butter, and sugar.

1¼ cup millet flour
1 cup whole-wheat pastry flour
1½ teaspoons baking powder
½ teaspoon baking soda
½ teaspoon salt
½ lb. butter
⅔ cup maple syrup
6 eggs separated (See Separating Eggs in the Maple
    Pecan Muffins recipe)
1 teaspoon vanilla extract

1. Sift flours, baking powder, soda and salt together.

2. Cream butter with a pastry cutter or electric mixer. Whisk in maple syrup, egg yolks, and vanilla until well mixed. Butter will be lumpy.

3. Add flour mixture in stages, a cupful at a time. Mix just until combined. Do not over mix.

4. In a separate bowl use an electric mixer to whip egg whites until stiff peaks form. Gently fold into batter. Pour batter into a loaf pan lined with lightly buttered wax paper. Bake at 350°F for 1 hour.

❧ STRAWBERRY UPSIDE-DOWN TOFU CAKE ☙

1 cup strawberries, sliced
2 one-pound blocks tofu
3/4 cup maple syrup
1 tablespoon almond butter
1/2 teaspoon vanilla

Topping
1/8 teaspoon salt
1/4 cup chopped almonds
1 cup kamut, bran, or other flakes cereal
1 tablespoon maple syrup
1 teaspoon nut oil or unsalted melted butter

1. Preheat oven to 350°F.

2. Steam tofu blocks in a tightly covered pot over boiling water for five minutes. Generously butter an 8 x 8-inch baking pan.

3. Using a food processor blend tofu, maple syrup, almond butter and vanilla until well pureed. You may need to do this in two stages if your food processor is small. Line baking dish bottom with strawberry slices. Spread tofu mixture on top of strawberries using a rubber spatula to spread to the edges of pan.

4. Combine topping ingredients together in a bowl stirring with a metal spoon to crush cereal flakes. Spread over top of tofu.

5. Bake for 30 minutes. Allow to cool before eating.

❦ WHOLE GRAIN PIE CRUST ❧

(Makes crust for 2 open-faced pies or one covered pie.)

Pie crusts are not really that tricky, but they take time and perseverance. This recipe is well worth it. Make certain that all of your ingredients are cold. While cold butter is harder to work with, small pieces of butter left in the dough make the crust flakier. The glaze recipe is optional for a covered pie.

> 1 cup whole-wheat pastry flour
> 1 cup barley flour
> 1 teaspoon salt
> $\frac{1}{4}$ lb. butter (1 stick)
> 3 tablespoons maple syrup
> 1 to 2 tablespoons ice water

1. Sift both flours and the salt into a large mixing bowl. Cut in butter using a pastry cutter or cube butter before mixing in and use a butter knife to incorporate. Mix until the mixture is crumbly and there are no clumps of butter larger than the size of a pea.

2. Using a fork, gently stir in the maple syrup. Add ice water a spoonful at a time, mixing dough with hands just until dough sticks together. Knead slightly, forming dough into a ball. Cut ball in half and form into two balls. Return one ball to mixing bowl and refrigerate until ready to roll out. At this point you can wrap dough in plastic and freeze indefinitely.

3. Place one ball of dough between two pieces of wax paper. Flatten by hand and begin to roll into a circle with a rolling pin. Roll to about $\frac{1}{8}$-inch thickness. Check width of crust against pie pan by laying pan in center of crust. Crust should extend about 2 inches over pan edges.

4. Remove top piece of wax paper. Place pie pan upside down in the center of crust and flip. Gently lay crust into pie pan removing wax paper. Avoid stretching the dough or the crust will shrink while baking. Trim overhanging edges to about 1 inch. Any holes in the crust bottom can be filled by pressing in a small piece of trimming. Fold extra dough over on top of itself and scrimp the edges together with your fingers. If you are making a pie with a top crust, do not crimp edges and follow the directions for a top crust below.

5. For a pie with no top crust, prick crust bottom and sides 20 to 30 times with a fork to prevent bubbles from forming during baking. Bake crust at 400°F for 15 minutes until browned. Fill according to pie recipe.

6. If making a pie with a top crust, fill according to pie recipe and follow top crust directions below.

7. Top crust: Roll out top crust as with bottom to about ⅛-inch thickness.

8. Brush a little water onto edges of previously filled bottom crust.

9. Remove top piece of wax paper, carefully lift crust with bottom piece of wax paper and flip onto pie. Remove paper and trim leaving a generous inch of crust around the edge. Fold bottom crust over top and crimp using moist fingers, if necessary, to seal any holes. You may need to move extra crust from one spot to fill in a thinner spot. Be generous with the crust.

Glaze for top crust:
1 egg yolk
½ teaspoon maple syrup
½ teaspoon milk

1. Whisk glaze ingredients together. Brush glaze over top of pie paying special attention to edges.

2. Cut three lines or other shape into top crust to allow steam to escape. Brush crust with pie crust glaze and bake according to pie recipe.

✥ EVERYBODY-LOVES-YOU APPLE PIE ✥

1 pie crust recipe or two store-bought frozen whole
    grain crusts
7 to 8 Granny Smith apples, or other cooking apples
Zest of $\frac{1}{2}$ lemon
2 tablespoons arrowroot powder
$\frac{1}{3}$ cup maple syrup
2 tablespoons melted butter

1. Preheat oven to 350°F.
2. Peel and core apples. Chop into $\frac{1}{4}$-inch thick slices.
3. Roll out bottom crust to recipe directions and line 9-inch pie pan.
4. Toss together the apples, lemon zest and arrowroot. Pour in the maple syrup and melted butter and toss coating all the apples, separating slices by hand if necessary.
5. Spoon filling into bottom crust, spreading it to the edges and filling any holes with apples. It may seem as if you have too many apples but stuff them all in there anyway. Apples will shrink while baking.
6. Follow crust recipe for top crust. Or, remove defrosted, store-bought crust from its pan. Lay crust over apples and trim edges to about 1 inch. Using wet fingers carefully fold bottom crust edges over top and crimp neatly. If you are using store-bought crust, seal the edges together with wet fingers or a fork. Use crust trimmings to seal any holes completely.
7. Slice a large (3 inches) vent in the top of the pie and two smaller (1 inch) side vents. Brush with glaze and bake in oven

1 hour until filling is bubbling. Place a cookie sheet on an oven rack below the pie rack to catch the inevitable apple juice drippings.

8. Allow pie to cool before slicing. Delicious!

⚜ LIP SMACKIN' BLACKBERRY PIE ⚜

Boysenberries, raspberries, or any other favorite berry can be substituted for the blackberries in this recipe. Frozen fruit is more readily available and works fine in this recipe. Pie should be thoroughly cool before slicing. Serve with a dollop of fresh whipped cream or vanilla yogurt.

½ pie crust recipe
4 cup fresh or frozen blackberries
2 tablespoons arrowroot powder
¾ cup maple syrup
1 tablespoon lemon juice

1. Preheat oven to 400°F.

2. Roll out and line an 8-inch pie pan with crust. Fold over excess dough and crimp the edges prettily. Using a fork, generously prick crust bottom and sides to allow vents for steam to escape. Bake 10 minutes.

3. Meanwhile, combine maple syrup and lemon juice in a small bowl. Whisk in arrowroot powder a little at a time until there are no clumps. Place berries and maple syrup mixture into a saucepan and warm slowly over medium heat. Stir frequently and remove from heat when mixture begins to simmer. Mixture will have thickened. Pour into pre-baked pie crust using a heat-resistant rubber spatula to scrape the sides of pan.

4. Turn oven temperature down to 350°F and bake pie 30 minutes. Remove and allow to cool completely or refrigerate before serving.

PEACH-BERRY PIE

This delicious summertime pie can be enjoyed anytime of year with frozen fruit. Be sure to allow frozen fruit to defrost completely before using.

    1 pie crust recipe or 2 store-bought frozen whole grain crusts
    1 cup blueberries, strawberries, or blackberries
    4 cup sliced peaches
    1/4 cup maple syrup
    2 tablespoons arrowroot

1. Roll out bottom crust to pie crust directions and carefully line a 9-inch pie pan. If using store-bought crusts, allow them to defrost completely before using.

2. Gently toss together all of the filling ingredients, making sure the arrowroot doesn't lump up.

3. Spoon the filling into bottom crust spreading to edges. Follow pie crust directions for a top crust, or remove second store bought crust from its pan and lay on top of pie.

4. Using wet fingers carefully crimp edges together sealing completely.

5. Bake 40 to 45 minutes at 400°F.

6. Cool before serving.

PUMPKIN PIE

    1/3 cup raw wheat germ
    Butter
    2 cup pumpkin
    2 eggs (fertile, cage-free)
    1/4 cup Amazake (or light cream)
    1/2 cup rice beverage
    1/2 cup maple syrup

1 teaspoon vanilla
¼ cup raisins
¼ teaspoon sea salt
½ teaspoon cinnamon
¼ teaspoon ginger (fresh is best)
¼ teaspoon allspice
⅛ teaspoon cloves
2 teaspoons arrowroot starch
1 teaspoon dark rum (optional)
⅛ teaspoon Garam Masala (optional)

1. Butter a non-aluminum pie plate generously. Add raw wheat germ, and coat pie plate evenly.

2. Blend remaining ingredients until raisins are well blended. Pour filling into crust. Bake at 350°F for 1 hour.

❧ SOUTHERN PECAN PIE ☙

½ pie crust recipe
1 cup pecan halves or pieces
1½ cup barley malt
4 eggs
2 tablespoons whole-wheat flour
1 tablespoon butter
¼ teaspoon salt
½ teaspoon nutmeg

1. Preheat oven to 350°F.

2. Roll out pie crust and fit into pie pan folding edges over generously and pinching to hold with your fingers.

3. In a blender combine all ingredients except the pecans. Blend until frothy. Place pecans on bottom of pie shell and pour barley malt mixture over them being sure to wet all the pecans.

4. Bake 40 minutes until firm and golden.

19

Expanding Your Diet

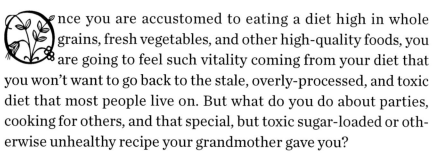

nce you are accustomed to eating a diet high in whole grains, fresh vegetables, and other high-quality foods, you are going to feel such vitality coming from your diet that you won't want to go back to the stale, overly-processed, and toxic diet that most people live on. But what do you do about parties, cooking for others, and that special, but toxic sugar-loaded or otherwise unhealthy recipe your grandmother gave you?

Let me say that I speak from experience here. I have spent over thirty years cooking for family and guests who thought that they were eating "gourmet food" instead of "health food." The real trick is to care enough about yourself and your family to select only the highest quality ingredients and prepare them with love.

If you serve guests a meal with baked fish, Dr. Huntley's Foolproof Recipe for Delicious Brown Rice, and a fresh salad with Incredible Salad Dressing, they are not going to know this is a special diet. If you are invited over to a friend's house, be honest. Tell him or her that you are on a special diet and discuss the menu. There will probably be some things you can eat. It's always a good idea to offer to bring dessert.

Desserts are usually the weak point for most people at parties. Honestly, if I'm invited to a big party, I usually eat before I go, nibble on things that don't look too toxic, and enjoy the company.

Now, about that killer recipe from your grandmother: I have some of them, too, but I have found ways to create healthier food by following these steps:

1. Substitute whole grain flours for white flour. You can find whole-wheat pastry flour, which is lighter than regular whole-wheat flour. Barley flour makes great pancakes. Millet flour is wonderful in pound cake. Try a mixture of flours to lighten up a cake recipe. To make a cake come out extra light, separate the eggs, beat the whites until stiff, and fold in the whites as the last step.

2. Substitute maple syrup as a sweetener. This is easy for recipes that use honey or molasses, but it gets a little trickier when substituting for sugar. Cut down the amount of water, milk, or other liquid in the recipe by the amount of maple syrup you add, but you may have to adjust that a little by trial and error. Cookies are a real problem, and you may have to stick to recipes that contain nut butters, which blend with the maple syrup to give the dough a more solid consistency. Do not try to use maple syrup in making yeast breads. Maple syrup kills fungi, so it will kill the yeast and the bread won't rise. (I speak from experience.) Of course, the yeast digests the sugar as it grows and makes the bread rise, so you don't have to worry about excess sugar in the bread.

3. Substitute lemon juice for vinegar almost anywhere. Vinegar is not good for people with fungal problems, which includes almost everyone.

Over time, you will become more creative as you practice the fine art of cooking healthy food for yourself, your family, and your friends.

20

Take Control of Your Health

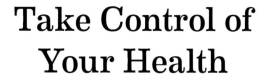

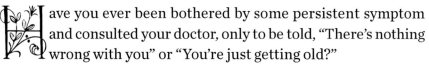ave you ever been bothered by some persistent symptom and consulted your doctor, only to be told, "There's nothing wrong with you" or "You're just getting old?"

Have you been concerned because of a health problem that runs in your family and you have no way of knowing whether your diet is preventing you from getting ill or making it more certain that you will?

Have you wished that you had some way to tell which diet is optimum for *you*?

If your answer is "Yes" to any of these questions, then I have good news. You are in possession of a fine-tuned "instrument" that can enable you to determine exactly what foods are the right ones for you to eat at any given time!

Your instrument is probably not in good working order. It might need cleaning and possibly some repairs, but it is the best instrument ever made for determining the right diet for you.

This instrument is your sense of smell and taste!

Watch an animal when it is not feeling well. It will be "off its feed." It may go out and eat certain grasses or weeds, and sometimes this will work to get it over the problem. How does it determine which foods it needs to eat in order to cure itself? Well, apparently these foods taste good at the time the animal needs them. This system could work for you, except that you have likely poisoned your sensory mechanisms.

A diet that is high in fats, sugars, salt, and artificial chemicals actually destroys the sensory nerve endings of the organs of smell and taste. It does damage to the eye and ear receptors, too. Natural foods no longer stimulate these nerves properly after this damage, so the temptation is to add more powerful stimulants to the food to create some effect on the sense of taste, such as hot peppers or more sugar. The damage just builds up. Fortunately, this damage is reversible. The nerve endings can repair themselves if they are given respite from the chemical barrage and good nutrition.

The bad news is that it may take several months of what seems like a severely bland diet to get your self-healing mechanisms in working order, although taking supplements can shorten your recovery time.

But do you like the idea that what tastes delicious to you is the very thing that can nourish and help repair your body? Good—then get to work!

References

Let's Eat Right to Keep Fit by Adelle Davis; Signet Books; Revised edition, 1970

The Rockefeller File by Gary Allen; 76 Press, 1976

Are you a target for elimination: An inside look at the AMA conspiracy against chiropractic and the wholistic healing arts by P.J. Lisa; International Institute of Natural Health Sciences; 1984

Stalking the Wild Asparagus (Deluxe Edition, 2005) by Euell Gibbons; Alan Cup Hood & Co., Inc.; (First Edition, 1962)

Eat Right 4 Your Type: the Individualized Diet Solution to Staying Healthy, Living Longer, & Achieving Your Ideal Weight by Dr. Peter D'Adamo and Catherine Whitney; Berkley; 1st Edition; 1996. Note: We have included this reference because Dr. Huntley often suggested diets for her clients based on their blood type.

Field of Greens: New Vegetarian Recipes From the Celebrated Greens Restaurant by Annie Somerville; Bantam Books, New York, N.Y.; 1993

Mad Cowboy: Plain Truth from the Cattle Rancher Who Won't Eat Meat by Howard Lyman; Scribner, New York, N.Y.; 2001

http://www.cancertutor.com/budwig

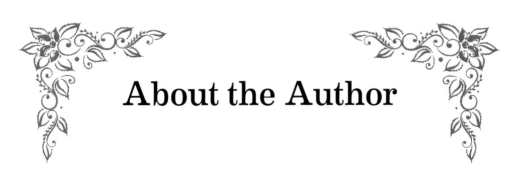

About the Author

Elizabeth Huntley, PhD was born on May 19, 1940 in Louisiana, Missouri.

From 1981 until 2007, when she retired from private practice as a nutritionist, Elizabeth helped thousands of people improve their health using proper diet, supplements, pure water, and other natural healing modalities.

Elizabeth Huntley is a highly talented medical intuitive. In addition to her natural-born diagnostic skills, her consultations are based on the education she received from these institutions:

Swarthmore College, BA Physics
Brown University, MSC Biology
Brown University, PhD Biological and Medical Sciences

Over the course of her career as a practicing nutritionist, Elizabeth Huntley often suggested supplements from Standard Process Labs to her patients. She also used a radionics device called the "SE 5" to help her arrive at the most accurate diagnosis quickly—often for people living at a distance who were unable to visit her in person.

Elizabeth Huntley currently resides in Medford, Oregon.

Elizabeth can be contacted by e-mail to
editor@mind.net
or by contacting Robert D. Reed Publishers

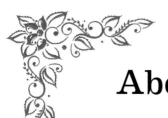

About the Editor

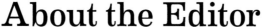

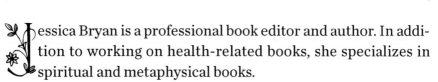

essica Bryan is a professional book editor and author. In addition to working on health-related books, she specializes in spiritual and metaphysical books.

She lives in Southern Oregon with Tom Clunie D.C., who offered valuable suggestions during the editing of Elizabeth Huntley's book.

Jessica can be reached by e-mail at
editor@mind.net
or telephone: 541-708-0729.
On the web: www.oregoneditor.wordpress.com